# Erectile Dysfunction

## A Complete Guide to Manage Erectile Dysfunction

What Is Erectile Dysfunction, Symptoms, Causes, Risks, Complications, Common Misconceptions, Medical and Natural Treatments All Included!

By: Frederick Earlstein

# Foreword

Erectile dysfunction is something that every man will have to deal with at some time in his life for some reason or other. It's worrying from a man's point of view when this happens, though is certainly nothing that he needs to worry too much about because this book has enough information to help.

Included inside this book's first section is about understanding erection and erectile dysfunction. It also contains information about its causes, symptoms, risks, and complications.

The Second section will talk about the main underlying health conditions, and lifestyle factors you should know about that are most likely to be causing erectile dysfunction.

The third section will discuss the common myths and misconceptions about erectile dysfunction.

The next section focuses on the medical treatments for erectile dysfunction.

The fifth section will cover how to cure erectile dysfunction naturally.

In the next part, you will learn how to have full and happy sex lives despite suffering from erectile dysfunction.

The seventh section will tackle how a sex therapist could help with erectile dysfunction and help you decide if you need one.

The last section will talk about how the lack of confidence is related to erectile dysfunction. It will also discuss the ways how to increase your self-confidence.

Erectile dysfunction is a familiar condition among men, but it doesn't mean you can't do anything about it. Erectile dysfunction treatments need not be embarrassing or complicated. There are approaches and natural ways to overcome impotence.

Attempt these treatments and begin building your sexual self-confidence. You don't have to conceal your state. It can be treated, and you can have a healthy, happy sexual life. Everybody deserves it, and that includes you.

## Table of Contents

# Introduction

Did you know that about 25% of men aged 20-75 suffer from ED (erectile dysfunction)? According to the National Institute of Health, approximately 5% of all American men above the age of 40 suffer from ED while 15-25% of 65-year-old men experience ED long term. As you can see from the above statistics, ED is a very common problem. Additionally, statistics show that ED affects most men at one point or the other in their lives. This means that most men occasionally fail to achieve an erection for one reason or the other. However, it is important to point out that failure to achieve an erection less than 20% of the time i.e., 2 out of every 10 times you have sex, does not necessarily count as erectile dysfunction and therefore treatment in this case is not necessary. On the other hand, failure to achieve an erection 50% of the time i.e., 5 times out of every 10 times a man engages in sex, hints at an underlying problem, qualifies as ED, and requires treatment.

To most men, erectile dysfunction is a very embarrassing thing despite it being a medically diagnosed ailment. Part of the reason for this is the simple fact that most men consider an erection part of their manhood. Therefore, when a man cannot 'get it up' something inside him shifts and makes him feel less of a man. In this state, it is impossible for the man to have a trusting and lasting relationship with his wife or 'lady friend'. He may lash out, become cold and distant, or even break up the relationship altogether. Further, the fact that men, their penis and its problems is not a 'dinner-table' conversation does very little to help the situation. When most men discover they have ED, they keep mum about it and silently kill themselves over it.

This does not have to be the case. The penis and its problems is something any loving and trusting couple should discuss openly. Did you know that about 65% of all men on the globe are unhappy with their erection? This is according to a 2008 Better Sex Survey published in the Journal of Sexual Medicine. Despite these statistics, it should not surprise you to learn that most couples rarely talk about ED. Fortunately ED is a treatable ailment.

Before we can look at ED treatment and cure, we need to understand it. We shall do this by looking at the various facets of erectile dysfunction. Let us do that now.

# Chapter One: Understanding Erectile Dysfunction

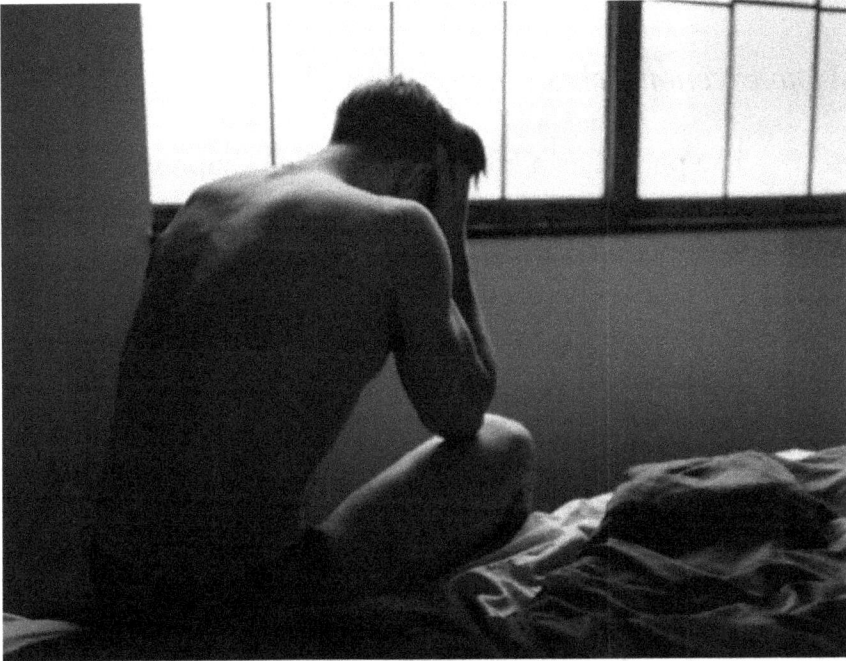

## *What Is An Erection?*

An erection is the process whereby a man's penis stands erect in order for him to make love or have sexual intercourse and easily penetrate his woman's vagina and ejaculate semen. Usually, erections take place in a healthy man when he is sexually aroused or sexually excited or stimulated. Sometimes, it happens when the man is touched sexually or if he sees a naked woman or girl live or her picture or thinks about having sex with someone. Sometimes, it occurs without thinking of sex or being touched when one wakes up or during the night and sometimes, it happens unexpectedly.

## *How Erection Takes Place/Happens?*

The penis has a banana or sausage shape with a duct or tube known as the "urethra" that run through the penis. Both the semen and urine passes through the urethra to get out of the body. The urethra is made up of tissue known as "the corpus spongiosum penis" this is a Latin word known as "body of the penis"

The penis has tissue that are close to the upper surface area (two cylindrical tissues) known as: corpora cavernosa penis (caves) and the other one is known as "corpus cavernosum" all these tissues have lots of blood vessels known as "arteries" that carries the blood.

Let's look at how erections take place now. Whenever a guy or man is sexually aroused or stimulated, which might arise as a result of a sexual touch which could be masturbation or touched by an opposite sex (woman) in a sexually way or when he sees or watch sexual pictures or pornography or a naked woman. Immediately, the nerves in the arteries of the two cylindrical tissues in the penis will cause a chemical known as nitric oxide to be released into the arteries which will compel it to dilate and be filled with blood. Now, all the tissues will now be filled with blood and the penis will become longer, larger, thicker, stronger and harder. Finally, the tissue known as 'corpora cavernosa' will press against the blood vessels known as 'veins' that helps in carrying of blood out of the penis and a valve will pop up to stops the urine from entering the urethra. This is why, only semen flows along the urethra and very difficult to urinate during erection.

Erections does not happen only through the above reasons as it can happen when one imagines he is having sex with someone or sees a naked person. In this type of situation, the man's brain sends a signal or message to the penis through the spinal cord and an erection will take place. The most important thing about the brain is the fact that it can stop erections even if you are touched in a sexual way.

Once you have an orgasm and ejaculation or you are not sexually aroused, your erections will come to an end and your penis will become small again. The time it will take for your erection to fall depends on the length and thickness of your penis.

## Types Of Erections?

Basically, there are two types of erections known as:

1. Erections when sleeping or morning glory or wood: erection when sleeping is also known as 'nocturnal penile tumescence' this is the type of erections that occurs by itself when you are sleeping and dreaming. This type of erection usually occurs when your bladder is filled with

urine which will lead to the pressing of your penis tissues and thus leading to an erection.

2. Unexpected erections or sudden or surprise (spontaneous) erection: this type of erection is common with teenagers and sometimes adult do experience this type of erections. This type of erection is an involuntary and is normal type of erection that can happen anytime at anywhere.

## What Are The Component Of Male Sexual Functions?

There are three (3) important components of male sexual functions which include:

1. Libido: this has to do with the desire or interest for sexual intercourse.
2. Erection: this has to do with the ability to have and keep erection for sexual intercourse.
3. Ejaculation: this is the last component that has to do with orgasm and releasing of semen.

## What is Erectile Dysfunction?

Erectile Dysfunction plagues men from all over the globe. It can be quite disturbing and causes issues in their social life, physical life, and even causes mental issues. In this section, you are going to learn what Erectile Dysfunction (ED) is. You will also learn what the causes are for ED.

Are you unsure of what Erectile Dysfunction really is? Quite simply ED is the inability to have or even keep an erection that is firm enough to engage in intercourse. It can also be referred to with the term, impotence. Erectile Dysfunction is not uncommon. There are numerous men that will experience Erectile Dysfunction for one reason or another throughout their lifetime. It could be caused by one or multiple reasons, which are covered later on in this chapter.

Not all of the sexual problems in men are caused by Erectile Dysfunction. There are other types that include:

- Delayed Ejaculation
- Absent Ejaculation
- Premature Ejaculation
- Lack of Sexual Interest

## Is Erectile Dysfunction Common?

There are over thirty million men in the United States of America alone that feel the effects of Erectile Dysfunction. This number was estimated by the National Institute of Diabetes and Digestive and Kidney Diseases, also referred to as NIDDK. The risk of Erectile Dysfunction increase as the man's age increases. Erectile Dysfunction affects 4% of all men that are in their 50s, but almost 17% of the men that are in their 60s. Over half of the men that are in their late 70s suffer from Erectile Dysfunction.

Even though the risks of Erectile Dysfunction increase as the age does, Erectile Dysfunction may not be inevitable when aging. It can be more difficult to actually get an erection as the man ages; however, it does not mean that the man will develop Erectile Dysfunction. Over all, the healthier the man is, the better his sexual function will be.

## How does a male get the erection?

When the blood flow to the man's penis increases, the penis will firm and/or grow. This is called an erection. The blood flow is typically stimulated by sexual arousal from thoughts or even direct contact to their penis. Once a man is sexually aroused, the muscles in their penis will relax. The relaxation allows the blood to flow through his penile arteries. This blood will fill two chambers that are inside his penis. They are called the corpora cavernosa. As these chambers fill with the blood, the penis will then grow rigid. The erection will end once the muscles contract and the accumulated blood flows out through the penile veins.

Erectile Dysfunction may occur from problems at any stage of the process. For an example, the penile arteries could be too damaged in order to open up properly to allow blood flow.

## *Causes of Erectile Dysfunction*

There are so many different causes for Erectile Dysfunction. The man can have one or more issues that can cause this issue. Sexual arousal is definitely a complex process that involves the man's brain, emotions, hormones, muscles, nerves, and even his blood vessels. This condition can be related to a medical issue, or even an emotional issue.

At times, a combination of the psychological and the physical issues will cause Erectile Dysfunction. For example, if the man has a minor physical issue that slows his sexual response, it may cause some anxiety on the subject of maintaining an erection. The anxiety will lead to or even worsen Erectile Dysfunction.

**Physical Causes**

In typical cases, the Erectile Dysfunction issue is brought on by physical problems. Here is a list of common physical conditions that will cause Erectile Dysfunction.

- Clogged Blood Vessels
- Heart disease
- High Blood Pressure
- High Cholesterol
- Obesity
- Diabetes
- Metabolic Syndrome
- Multiple Sclerosis
- Parkinson's Disease
- Peyronie's Disease
- Use of Tobacco
- Prescription Medicines
- Alcohol

- Insomnia and Other Sleeping Disorders
- Surgeries
- Injuries
- Treatments for Prostate Cancer

**Psychological Causes**

The brain plays a very large role in triggering different physical events that will cause an erection. It starts with the feelings of the man. There are a numerous amount of aspects that can interfere with his sexual feelings and can cause or even worsen Erectile Dysfunction. These typical causes include:

- Depression
- Anxiety
- Other Mental Health Problems
- High Level of Stress
- Problems in their Relationship
- Poor Communication with his Partner
- Other Life Stresses
- 

## *Erectile Dysfunction Symptoms and Risk*

Now that you know what Erectile Dysfunction is; in this section you will learn what the symptoms and the risks are with this condition. This is one of the first steps in battling Erectile Dysfunction.

## Signs and Symptoms of Erectile Dysfunction

The signs and the symptoms are the same thing when is comes to this disorder. Just as the description of Erectile Dysfunction states, this is known to be an issue when the man is unable to get or maintain an erection.

## Risk Factors of Erectile Dysfunction

As a man gets older, the erections may take a bit longer to develop and may not be as firm as it needs to be for intercourse. The man may need a more direct touch to the penis to maintain the erection. This may indicate an underlying health problem or can be a result of a mediation being taken. There are other aspects that can raise the risk of Erectile Dysfunction.

- *Medical Problems*: In most cases when it comes to medical issues that cause Erectile Dysfunction, it is typically diabetes or heart problems.

- *Obesity*: This is a normal cause for Erectile Dysfunction.

- *Smoking*: Tobacco restricts the blood flow to your veins and arteries. Over some time it can cause a lot of chronic health conditions that will also lead to Erectile Dysfunction.

- *Specific Medical Treatments*: There are treatments that will cause Erectile Dysfunction. One treatment is for prostate surgery or even radiation treatment for different types of cancer.

- *Injuries*: There are different injuries that can cause Erectile Dysfunction. If there is damage to nerves or to the arteries that control an erection, then the male will be subjected to Erectile Dysfunction.

- *Prescribed Medications*: There are medicines that will cause this issue. Medications like antidepressants, high blood pressure medicine, and antihistamines can cause Erectile Dysfunction. Some others include pain medicine and prostate medicines.

- *Psychological Issues*: Stress, depression, and even anxiety can cause Erectile Dysfunction.

- *Drug Use and Alcohol Use*: These items can cause issues with muscles, mental condition, and nerves, among other aspects of getting an erection.

- *Bicycling*: Prolonged bicycling can cause the nerves to become compressed and will affect the blood flow to a man's penis. It can lead to a temporary issue or even a permanent issue.

## The Outlook of Erectile Dysfunction

Erectile Dysfunction can be helped or treated by a range of different treatments or techniques. It ranges from drugs, natural remedies, to surgery. Depending on the condition that is causing the Erectile Dysfunction treatments will vary.

## Complications of Erectile Dysfunction

There are, of course, complications due to Erectile Dysfunction. They are psychological though. Here is a list of issues that are caused by Erectile Dysfunction.

- Unsatisfied Sexually
- Stress from Condition
- Anxiety form Condition
- Embarrassment
- Low Self Esteem
- Problems in Relationship
- Inability to Impregnate Partner

# Chapter Two: Causes of Erectile Dysfunction

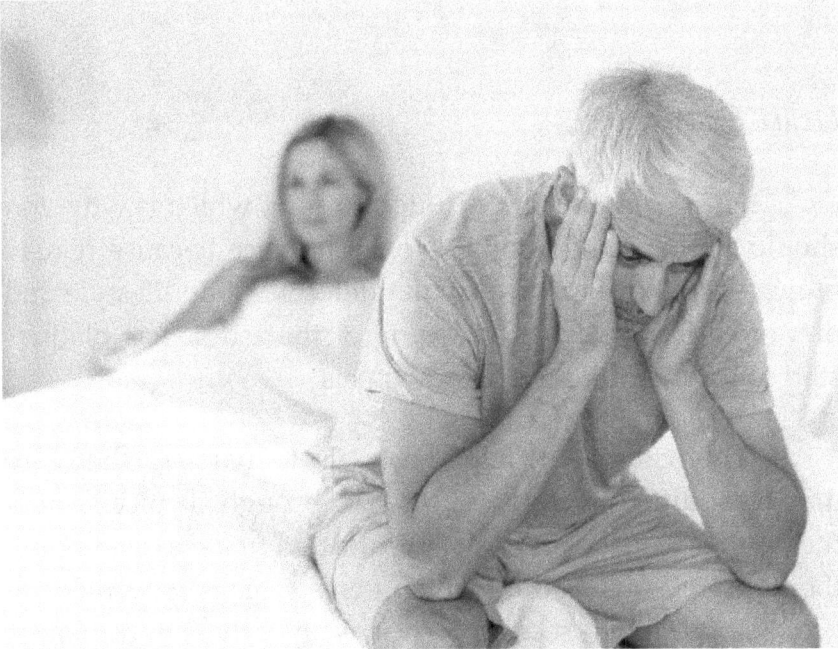

There are several main causes of erectile dysfunction. In order to address your impotence, it is important to figure out the root cause of the problem first, so you can cure it for good.

Most men are embarrassed to inform their doctors about erectile dysfunction, and even if they do, they are hoping for a simple cure in the form of a blue pill. This is not how this works. More often than not, your doctor will insist on a complete diagnosis to ensure that there are no serious health risks that could be the root cause of your condition

Here are the main underlying health conditions and lifestyle factors you should know about that most likely to be causing your ED:

## Heart Disease

Heart disease can be tough to spot, which is why you should probably be thankful for impotence because it may indicate you have cardiovascular defects. A bad lifestyle and diet often leads to the hardening of the arteries as plaques start to form around the blood vessels.

This causes the blood vessels to narrow, therefore making it difficult for blood to pass through. Typically, it is the smaller blood vessels that get affected first – case in point: the blood vessels leading to the penis. This is why medical professionals often see impotence as an early sign of plaque buildup in the blood vessels, which can cause fatal harm if left alone.

## Diabetes

Diabetes is one of those health problems that can negatively affect the whole body. Due to the elevated levels of sugar in their body, men with diabetes may have damaged nerves and blood vessels attributed with maintaining an erection. That said, men with diabetes may have the urge to have sex but unable to get an erection or even if they do, it is not firm enough for penetration.

Typically, diabetes-caused erectile dysfunction is treated with medications as well as lifestyle changes to minimize the damage caused by the problem. However, medications like Viagra® may not be an option if the person also suffers from heart problems, a common condition that comes with diabetes.

## Obesity

There's some information circulating that fat men actually last longer in bed for the simple fact that they have more sugar to burn. Although this might be slightly true, there's a small line separating sexual stamina and impotence. You'll find that adding on more weight can actually lead to erectile dysfunction because the body suddenly slows its testosterone production, hence the difficulty in maintaining an arousal.

That's just a small part of the overall problem – obesity can also trigger other health problems such as hypertension, diabetes, and cardiovascular problems – all of which are capable of damaging the blood vessels.

## Prostate Problems

Prostate problems include inability to urinate, difficulty while urinating, sometimes having sudden urges to empty their bladder too often or not often enough. Although impotence is not a side effect of the condition, it's been noted that treatments for prostate problems can cause erectile dysfunction. This is true for both surgery and pill treatments.

## Alcohol

Alcohol is another common cause of erectile dysfunction, starting with temporary erection problems and eventually leading to a long-term condition. This is because alcohol reduces blood flow to the brain as well as to the penis. Men who drink alcohol are also slower to obtain an erection and more often than not, the orgasm is weak.

Long-term impotence is possible for males who drink spirits on a chronic basis or those largely dependent on alcohol. Loss of sexual desire and premature ejaculation are also some side effects of drinking too much alcohol.

## Smoking

Another good reason to quit smoking is the fact that it actually helps you achieve thicker, firmer, and longer-lasting erections. Again, the culprit here is the damage to the blood vessels. Smoking tends to interfere with blood flow, especially in heavy smokers. However, you might not realize just how big an impact this has on your body.

A study shows that non-smokers experienced faster arousal compared to smoking counterparts – as much as 5 times faster in reaching full penile thickness. Not only that, but they've also managed to hold longer during sex, which means that their partners are fully satisfied with the session. Fortunately, smoking doesn't cause extensive damage. Unless you've been smoking obsessively for the past years, quitting this vice can help restore the thickness and hardness of your penis.

## Processed Foods

Shockingly, erectile dysfunction is beginning to appear in men in their early 20's. The American diet is loaded with trans fats, sugars starches and preservatives that's being consumed in excess is taking its toll on young adults.

Did you know that the average American body is so incredibly toxic that it would take 7 years longer to fully decompose an American body than then a corpse from most other countries and it has nothing to with our embalming techniques.

It's also widely acknowledged that impotence is caused by a diet high in trans fats, sugars and starchy foods that can block the blood flow that causes erections. Ironically, these are the same foods causing all the medical conditions stated above. It's become increasingly clear that erectile dysfunction is no longer a condition just related to age.

## Porn Induced ED

Evidence increasingly suggests that porn is responsible for erectile dysfunction in 15-20% of men in their early 20's. A survey of 28,000 young Italian men reported that excessive porn watching lowered men's libido and was responsible for their inability to get an erection.

Excessive porn can desensitize men to sex so that they can no longer get excited by real, everyday sexual encounters. It can also lead to unrealistic expectations that raise a man's tolerance for sex.

## Pre-Workout Supplements

It's worth mentioning, although there have been no official studies, that there is a growing number of men using pre-workout supplements who complain of erectile dysfunction after taking them. Many brands contain heavy stimulants that are much worse on your health than caffeine containing stimulants like 1,3 Dimethyl, which is a potent vasoconstrictor.

Vasoconstrictors narrow blood vessels and will reduce blood flow to the penis. Warning: Never take Viagra when you are using a product that contains vasoconstrictors.

## Medications

Although it's not discussed as much as it should be, both prescription and over the counter medications are among the most common causes of ED. Research shows that prescription drugs are responsible for up to 1 of out of every 4 cases of erectile dysfunction and this estimate may be an understatement of the real numbers.

- Antidepressants such as Prozac, Zoloft, and Lexapro are known causes of ED. According to Medscape, 60% of people taking anti-depressants experience ED. Although experts are unsure exactly how it is related, it is suspected that these drugs have an effect on our neurotransmitters such as serotonin, norepinephrine, and dopamine that affect our feelings of well-being.

- High Blood Pressure Medication While high blood pressure itself can cause ED, research shows that many of the medications used to treat high blood pressure can also cause ED, making the problem two-fold. They can cause decreased blood flow to the penis which can interfere with erections. Studies show that 3 types of blood-pressure drugs — diuretics (or "water pills"), alpha-blockers, and beta-blockers have the highest incidence of sexual interference.

- Cholesterol Lowering Medication- Research has shown that by lowering cholesterol, a building block of hormones, cholesterol medications (statins) disrupt the production of testosterone, estrogen and other sex hormones.

- Allergy Medication  Can cause a temporary form of erectile dysfunction (ED). Though it's not exactly clear how it causes ED, it is thought that it could change the way a man's nervous systems reacts to stimulation around his penis. Most times it's temporary and sensation returns gradually after stopping use.

- Heartburn Medication- Drugs such as Zantac and Pepcid that are used to treat gastrointestinal disorders can cause ED when taken in high doses. Tagament is also likely to cause men sexual difficulty and interestingly enough, is also reported to cause breast growth.

# Chapter Three: Common Myths and Misconceptions

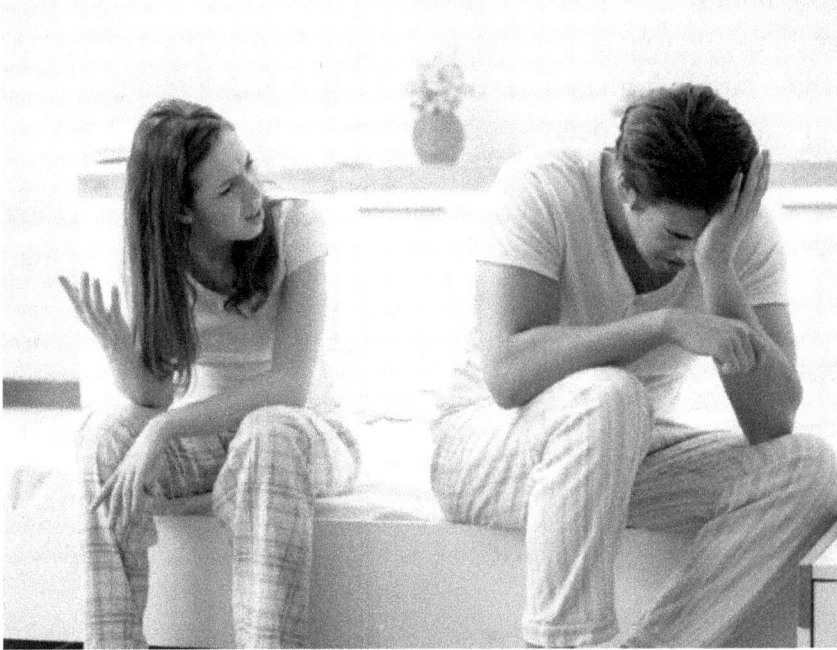

There are many beliefs going on around what causes erectile dysfunctions – some are myths and some are not exactly mythical. So, which is which? In this chapter, we'll take a look at some of the most common beliefs about erectile dysfunction and their veracity.

## *Wearing Tight Underwear Causes Erectile Dysfunction*

This is a common myth that you frequently hear about. However, it is completely untrue. It is a misconception that is based off of another unrelated medical fact. This fact is that wearing tight underwear keeps testicles too close to the body, which results in higher heat levels than is optimal for sperm production. This results in infertility. However, this infertility and erectile dysfunction are two completely different things. If you suffer from erectile dysfunction, it is unlikely that your sperm count has been affected by this.

Additionally, if you are suffering from infertility, then you probably won't have any difficulties getting erect because infertility has nothing to do with the amount of blood that flows into your groin. Thus, wearing tight underwear will not cause erectile dysfunction.

## Erectile Dysfunction Means You Don't Like Your Partner

A common source of stress for men with erectile dysfunction is that their inability to get erect means that they do not love their wives, girlfriends or partners. This ends up causing more stress which further exacerbates the erectile dysfunction.

However, there is absolutely no reason to think this way about your partner. Your erectile dysfunction is the result of low blood flow to your penis or a low amount of testosterone in your bloodstream. It has nothing to do with how attractive your partner is, or how much you love him or her. Worrying about something like this will only make your erectile dysfunction worse, so it is better to avoid the topic altogether. If you really feel as if this is the case, talk to your therapist about it. They will be able to at least talk you through the emotions that you are feeling.

## *Erectile Dysfunction becomes Naturally Inevitable with Age*

A common fear that a lot of men have is that when they get old, they are going to end up suffering from erectile dysfunction. This is because there is a tendency among older men to get this sexual dysfunction.

As a result, men who cross their mid-forties start to stress out about whether they are going to start suffering from this dysfunction or not. Ironically, this stress ends up causing erectile dysfunction, which further proves the misconception that as you get older you will definitely get erectile dysfunction. Erectile dysfunction is similar to arthritis or cancer. These things are not inevitable as you grow older, they just become more likely. As long as you lead a healthy lifestyle and get adequate amounts of exercise, you are never going to have to worry about erectile dysfunction.

## *Erectile Dysfunction is Abnormal among Young People*

Another common cause of stress for men erectile dysfunction only happens to older men. Getting it while you are young is a sign that you are not sexually virile, or are just deficient in some way.

On the contrary, erectile dysfunction is common among men of every age. If you are leading an unhealthy lifestyle, chances are you are going to end up suffering from erectile dysfunction. It is not a sign that you are somehow sexually inferior, you just need to change some of your habits and you will be absolutely fine. As has been mentioned before, erectile dysfunction is definitely more prevalent among older men. However, just because it is somewhat uncommon among younger men does not mean that you are any less of a man for having it. Don't stress yourself out over it, just take it as natural part of life and get the therapy you need.

## The Best Way to Treat Erectile Dysfunction is by Using Medicine

Most people tend to think that if they suffer erectile dysfunction popping a Viagra is the best way to ensure that you don't have to deal with erectile dysfunction any longer. While medicines are effective at assuaging the symptoms of erectile dysfunction, they aren't even the first things doctors recommend in order to get over erectile dysfunction. The first step to getting over erectile dysfunction is altering your lifestyle, taking exercise and following a better diet. If you apply these principles to your life, you will get over your erectile dysfunction without too much struggle.

It is only in more serious cases where doctors start to prescribe medicines, as in such situations it is better to take the medicine and suffer from the side effects rather than not take the medicine at all. Hence, medicine is not the best way to combat erectile dysfunctions, diet and exercise is.

## *Erectile Dysfunction is All in Your Head*

While it is true that in most of the cases where erectile dysfunction has become a problem, the main issue lies with anxiety and social stress, it is a misconception that erectile dysfunction can only ever be caused by stress and other such psychological issues. Erectile dysfunction is also caused by a number of physiological problems as well. Low testosterone levels, kidney issues, fat that is blocking blood flow to that part of your body, all of these are legitimate issues that can cause erectile dysfunction.

Hence, if you are suffering from erectile dysfunction, don't automatically assume that it is being caused by your psyche. Doing so might just end up putting more pressure on you when you are unable to get over your sexual dysfunction through therapy and the like.

## *Erectile Dysfunction Can't be Caused by Riding a Bike*

This is one of those rare occasions where a misconception about something not causing erectile dysfunction turns out to be false. Riding a bike is widely considered to be a safe activity that can never cause erectile dysfunction. This is because there are a lot of rumors that go around about erectile dysfunction and none of them appear to be true.

With biking however, the rumor actually is true. By cycling a lot, you put pressure on your groin and restrict blood flow in that area. As a result, the blood vessels get damaged, leading to erectile dysfunction.

# Chapter Four: Medical Treatments for Erectile Dysfunction

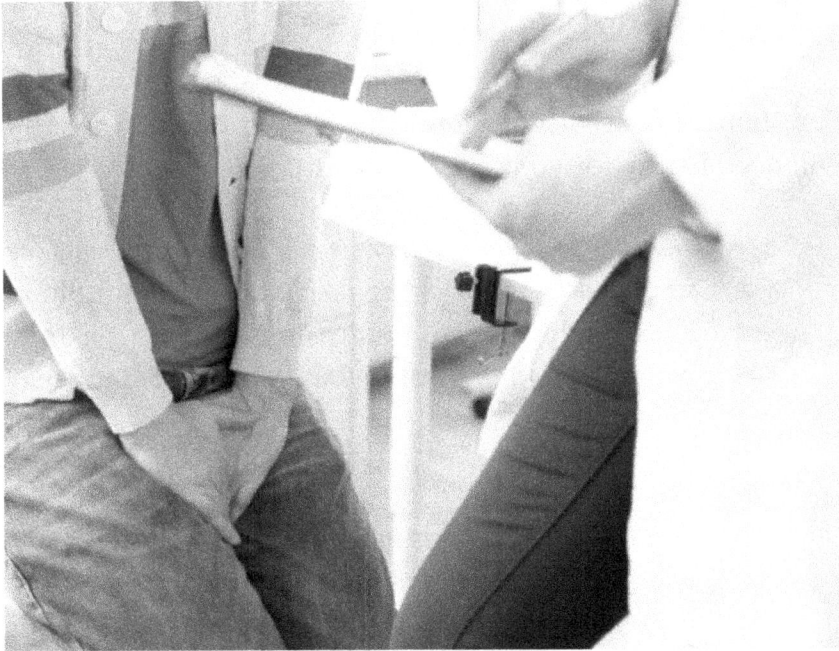

In this chapter, you will learn the information that you need from setting up the appointment to seeing your doctor and preparing for what happens in the medical world to treat those with Erectile Dysfunction. At times the medical way is the last resort. Most doctors will offer natural remedies before going to medical aids like medication or surgery.

## Prepare for the Appointment

You will more than likely begin with your family doctor or even a general practitioner. It will depend on the causes for your Erectile Dysfunction. The doctor may suggest a specialist depending on the cause, or even send you to a doctor that specializes in genital problems.

## Before Your Appointment

Before you appointment there are aspects of your life you should make a list of. Here is a walk through of what you will need handy for your appointment.

- *Ask the receptionist if there is anything special you may need to do before or bring for the appointment.* Blood tests might need to be done and the doctor may need you to avoid eating before the appointment.

- *Write down symptoms that you have experienced.* This needs to include anything that may seem unrelated. It might just be the cause of your condition.

- *Make a list of important personal information.* This includes any life changes, large situations that may have brought on a tremendous amount of stress, or any other mental conditions that you may be facing.

- *Take your partner with you.* This may seem embarrassing, but your partner may be able to offer up additional information that you may have forgotten or have not thought of as being part of the problem.

- *List of questions you would like to ask the doctor.* We all do it, we plan on asking key questions, but once in the doctor's office we forget them. Make a list of questions that pop into your head so you do not forget to ask.

## Questions to Add to Your List for the Doctor

Here is a list of basic questions that you will need to ask the doctor during your visit.

- What is the likely cause of the problem?
- What are the other possible causes?
- What tests should be done?
- Does it seem temporary or permanent?
- What is the best treatment for you?
- What are the alternatives to a medical approach?
- How can it be managed with other health problems?
- Are there any restrictions?
- Should you see a specialist?
- What will this cost?
- Will the insurance cover treatments?
- Is there a generic form of medication that can be prescribed?
- Is there any printed material that you can read to help with the understanding of Erectile Dysfunction?

## Questions the Doctor May Ask

Here is a list of some questions that the doctor may ask you. There may be more or even less. The list is to help prepare you to answer the questions and have the information ready.

- What health concerns or other chronic issues do you have?
- Have you had other sexual issues?
- Do you have any changes in your sex drive?
- Are you able to masturbate?
- Do you get an erection with the help of your partner or when you are sleeping?
- Are there problems in the relationship?
- Is there a problem with your sex life?
- Does your partner have a sexual issue?
- Do you feel depressed, anxious, or under a tremendous amount of stress?
- Have you been diagnosed with any mental disorders?
- Are you on any type of medicine for mental issues or physical disorders?
- Do you only experience Erectile Dysfunction at specific time, some times, or every time?
- When was the first time you experienced this?
- Do you take any natural remedies for anything?
- Do you drink much alcohol?
- Do you take any drugs; illegally?
- What improves the symptoms for you?
- What worsens the symptoms for you?

## Tests for Erectile Dysfunction

For many of the men that go to the doctor for this condition, they will be physically examined and answer questions about their medical history. The doctor will then offer a recommended treatment for the condition. If the issue is linked to a chronic health condition or if the doctor suspects that there may be an underlying condition, then you may have to see a specialist that your doctor will put you into contact with. Here is a list of tests that you may need to have done for Erectile Dysfunction.

- *Physical Examination*: This can include an examination of the penis, the testicles, and checking the nerves for different sensations.

- *Blood Test*: You may need to give a blood sample to run through the lab. It will look for underlying conditions, heart disease, low testosterone, or diabetes.

- *Urine Test*: Just like the blood tests, the urine test will be used to offer any signs of diabetes or other health conditions that could be a cause of your condition.

- *Ultrasound*: This is a test that is performed by the specialist in their office. It will involve using a wand type of devices that is held over your blood vessels that give blood to your penis. It will create a video image that will allow the doctor to see if there are any blood flow issues in the veins. At times this test is partnered with an injection of different medications into your penis in order to stimulate the flow of blood.

- _Overnight Test_: There are some men that will have an erection while sleeping. They will not remember due to the fact that they were sleeping. One test is to do an overnight erection test. It will involve wrapping a device around the penis before going to bed. It will measure the amount and strength of an erection that has been achieved through the night. It will help determine if the Erectile Dysfunction is related to a physical cause or psychological cause.

- _Psychological Examination_: The doctor may ask a few different questions to screen for anxiety, depression, or other psychological causes of your Erectile Dysfunction.

## Diagnosis of Erectile Dysfunction

There is a range of tools that will help the doctor evaluate the situation with Erectile Dysfunction. The doctor will most likely perform a physical examination as well as blood tests and urine tests. They may also use a questionnaire about your sexual health to help them understand your personal problem more. Some of the specialized tests will include:

- Doppler Ultrasonography
- Dye Injection for Blood Flow Imaging
- Nocturnal Penile Erection Monitoring
- Magnetic Resonance Imaging – MRI

## *Drugs and Treatment*

The very first thing that the doctor will do is ensure that you are receiving the right treatment for any other health conditions that you may have that could be causing your Erectile Dysfunction. Depending on your cause and the severity of the Erectile Dysfunction or any other health conditions, you may have different treatment options available. The doctor will be able to explain any of the risks, as well as the benefits of all treatments that are offered to you. It will also depend on the preferences of your partner.

## Oral Medicines

There are oral medications that have shown successful when using them for Erectile Dysfunction treatments for many males. These include:

- Tadalafil (Cialis)
- Sildenafil (Viagra)

- Avanafil (Stendra)
- Vardenafil (Levitra, Staxyn)

All four of the medications help enhance the effects of the nitric oxide. It is a natural chemical that the body produces that helps relax the muscles in the male's penis. This will increase the flow of blood and will allow the male to obtain an erection in response to some sexual stimulation.

Taking one the pills will not automatically cause an erection. The man must still be stimulated sexually in order to get an erection. The stimulation is needed to cause the release of the nitric oxide from the penile nerves. These medicines will amplify the signal that allows the men to function normally. Oral Erectile Dysfunction medicines are not considered aphrodisiacs, they will not cause the male to become exited and they are not needed in the men who can get erections on their own.

The medication dosage will vary on duration of the medicine as well as its side effects. Possible side effects can include flushing, headaches, nasal congestion, backache, visual changes, and even upset stomach.

The doctor will consider your situation to help determine what medication is right for you. The medicines may not fix your problem immediately. You may need to work with the doctor to find the right one for you, as well as the ideal dosage.

Before you take medication for the Erectile Dysfunction, make sure you speak with your doctor.

Medication for your issue may not work and may be dangerous due to different health conditions. They can be dangerous if you:

- Take any nitrate drugs. These are commonly prescribed when a person has chest pain like nitroglycerin, isosorbide mononitrate, or isosorbide dinitrate.
- Have low blood pressure issues or uncontrolled high blood pressure.
- Have liver disease that is severe.
- Have kidney disease that needs dialysis.

## Other Types of Medications

There are other medications that can be prescribed for this issue.

- **Alprostadil Self Injection**: With this specific method, you may use a small needle to inject the alprostadil into the base or the side of the penis. In some situations a combination of medications may be used that may provide a synergistic effect that will make the erection firmer and with less pain. Each of the injections will typically cause erections that will last about an hour. The needle that is used is very fine and the pain caused by the injection is typically very little. The side effect can be a slight aching sensation. Bleeding may also occur in the urethra if you did not do the injection properly.

- **Alprostadil Urethral Suppository**: Alprostadil intraurethral therapy will involve putting a small alprostadil suppository inside the penis. There is a specific applicator that is put inside the penis that then pushes the suppository in the penile urethra. The erection will begin in about 10 minutes and will last for 30-60 minutes. The side effects can be bleeding, pain, and formation of some fibrous tissues inside the penis.

- **Testosterone Replacement**: There are some that have Erectile Dysfunction that may be complicated by levels of testosterone that is too low. In this case testosterone replacement treatment may be the best route when treating Erectile Dysfunction.

## Penis Surgery, Implants, and Pumps

If you find that you are not responding to the medication or have serious side effects, there are other options that the doctor may offer to you. These include:

- **Penis Surgery**: The surgery that is performed on the blood vessels. At times the blood vessels may become obstructed or leak causing the Erectile Dysfunction. If this is the case, then the doctor will perform a surgical repair. It may include vascular stenting or a bypass.

- **Penis Implants**: This specific treatment will involve putting a device into both sides of your penis. The implants will consist of semi-rigid rods or inflatable rods. The inflatable rods will allow you to control the erection by when and how long you have one. The semi-rigid rods will keep the penis firm, yet not bendable. The penile implants typically are not recommended until the other methods are unsuccessful.
- **Penis Pumps**: A penis pump is a type of vacuum that causes an erection. It is a hollow type tube with a battery powered or hand powered pump. The tube is put on the penis and then the pump is used to suck the air from the tube. It creates a type of vacuum that pulls the blood into the penis. Once the man has the erection, he is able to put a ring on the base of the penis to hold in the blood. This will keep the penis firm. The pump will then be removed from the penis. The erection normally lasts long enough for the man to participate in sexual activities, although the penis will feel cold to touch.

## Therapy

Couples therapy is one area where people tend to shy away from if it concerns matters of sex. However, there is a special form of therapy, called sex therapy, which you can use in order to get past your erectile dysfunction. This is useful mostly in situations where the erectile dysfunction is caused by mental blockages. Stress, anxiety, shame, all of these things are perfectly legitimate factors that can affect your sex life. Hence, if you are suffering from erectile dysfunction and cannot find anything wrong with your prostate, and indeed nothing else with your body is wrong, then sex therapy may be your best option.

When you attend sex therapy, you are going to discover something very important: one of the most important factors affecting you is the fight or flight response. This is an ancient facet of human psychology that stretches all the way back to when we were still prey, and there were predators out there that could chase us. When we would be in dangerous situation where our life was in peril, our body would fill us with adrenaline so that we may either fight the entity that is posing a danger to us or flee. In a fight or flight response, you would need your blood flow redirected to your brain, so that you can judge the situation and see what kind of response is best, your arms, so that you can fight the thing that is posing a danger to you if the need arises, and your legs so that you can run as fast as you can.

Since blood flow is being redirected to so many different parts of your body, there is none left for your penis. No one needs an erection when they are fighting a foe, or so the body thinks. The problem in the modern day and age that we live in is that we experience the same old fight or flight responses in much more mundane situations. An example of this would be when you are about to have sex. If you are inexperienced with sex or are, for whatever reason, self-conscious about the way you look, your body would feel the same rush it would have felt ten thousand years ago if it was faced with a predator.

As a result, a lot of the blood flow is redirected from your groin and taken to your arms and legs, as well as your brain. Since there is no blood flow, you will be unable to get an erection. By going to sex therapy, you are going to be able to understand this very important fact about erectile dysfunction. You can also use sex therapy to ascertain what your emotional state is. A lot of the time, your erectile dysfunction might be caused by you being depressed. It is very possible to be depressed without knowing it, but going to sex therapy will allow you to rationalize the way you feel, facilitating a much more stable emotional state.

Another area where sex therapy can help you is performance anxiety. The majority of the time, performance anxiety is needless. It is based on unrealistic expectations instilled in you by pornography. A significant minority is caused by genuine concerns such as premature ejaculation, which would end up causing you to get so stressed that you would no longer be able to get an erection. Both of these situations can be helped significantly by going to sex therapy.

You can talk out your fears with your counselor and get over them, thereby allowing you to get over your erectile dysfunction.

## Hormone Therapy

One of the causes of erectile dysfunction is a low amount of testosterone in the body. This is usually coupled with low libido as well, and can be addressed by using hormone therapy. Hormone therapy essentially involves injecting yourself with testosterone. You can also use gels and patches that you will place upon your skin, through which the testosterone will be absorbed into the blood stream.

Once you begin taking testosterone, you are going to start feeling an increased desire for sex. This will at least make you passionate enough to use some of the alternate techniques that have been discussed in the previous section. One problem here is that testosterone does not improve blood flow to the penis. If you are suffering from that particular type of erectile dysfunction, testosterone won't be able to help you.

Additionally, taking testosterone can result in some serious side effects. Acne is a guaranteed side effect of taking testosterone, but some more major side effects can include an unnatural growth of your breasts as well as enlargement of your prostate. Only take testosterone if it has been prescribed by a doctor. There are situations where taking it could result in adverse health effects, such as if you suffer from prostate problems.

## Shockwave Therapy

This is a rather extreme way that you can treat your erectile dysfunction. By using electroshock therapy, or shockwave therapy, you are going to essentially rearrange the away your body makes flood flow within it. It is a reprogramming of your blood vessels in a way, and can stimulate major blood flow to your penis in particular. This is because it facilitates a process called revascularization. Through this process, your body can re grow or repair damaged blood vessels. When this happens, blood flow is promoted and your body becomes better able to transport blood to that particular area.

This has only been used so far to treat people who are recovering from heart attacks. It has been used only in very controlled situations for people who were suffering extreme cases of erectile dysfunction. Hence, no side effects are known yet. This is still a very new therapy, and has not been made available to the public. However, within a few years shockwave therapy may just become the single best way for you to overcome your erectile dysfunction, and it is important that you know as much about it as you can before it comes to the open market.

## Gadgets

### Electrostimulation Devices

These devices are a great solution for men who do not want to take any kind of medical treatment for their erectile dysfunction. The great benefit of this solution is that it involves no major medication, and is in general just a more intense form of prostate massage. These devices look like little pencils with wider ends that are made of metal. All you really have to do is insert it into your anus and turn it on, after which an electric charge will begin to course through it and stimulate your prostate.

This is an excellent way to promote the health of your prostate gland. If you are looking to increase the amount of testosterone in your body, or if you want to experience more pleasurable orgasms by stimulating your prostate, you can use these devices to help you get the job done.

Electrostimulation is an incredibly effective way to solve the problem of erectile dysfunction. Since your prostate is getting so heavily stimulated, within a week or so of regular use you are going to have so much blood flowing there that you will be able to get incredible erections without much effort, decidedly solving your problem of erectile dysfunction. Electrostimulation is not the sole realm of these wands, however. There are rings that you can place around your cock that will get the job done as well. These rings send a mild current through your penis that will get you hard in a surprisingly short amount of time. As it turns out, electricity on your penis ends up promoting a great deal of blood flow.

You can also get electrolytic creams that will make it a lot easier for you to conduct electricity through your penis, as well as prevent the chance of getting rashes with having the ring on for so long. You can try using a combination of these two electrostimulation devices. Both of these devices being used concurrently is an excellent way to ensure a healthy supply of testosterone and a large and continuous blood supply to that part of your body.

## Cock Rings and Vacuum Pumps

By using a pump, you can create a vacuum of blood in your penis. This will result in a great deal of blood rushing back into your penis, thereby engorging the spongy tissue and making your penis rigid and erect. The problem here is that the blood invariably goes rushing back down into your body. In order to stop this, you can use a cock ring. Cock rings cut off blood supply to your penis, thereby making it impossible for your body to suck the blood that has rushed into it back out.

The only problem here is that the cock ring can only be used for about twenty minutes before it can start causing damage to your blood vessels in that part of your body. Hence, cock rings and vacuum pumps are a short-term solution that is to be used only when you are about to have sex.

# Chapter Five: Natural Treatments for Erectile Dysfunction

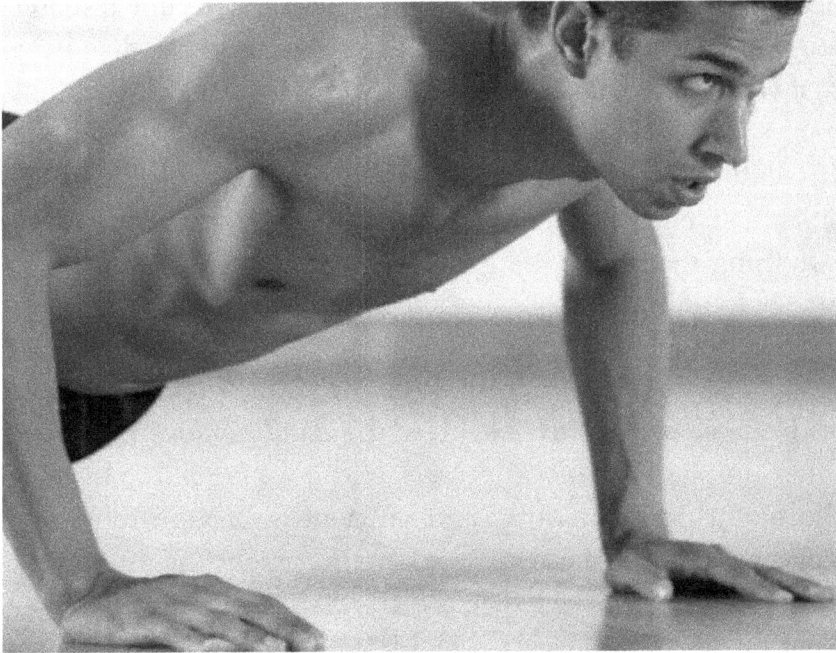

In most cases, erectile dysfunction can be attributed to a high-fat diet that can block the blood flow that causes erections. A lack of exercise or other reasons such as the wrong medication can leave men unaware of the impact small changes in their lives can have on their erectile dysfunction. The natural remedies in this section, in conjunction with sound medical advice can go some way in relieving erectile dysfunction.

## Exercise To Help Erectile Dysfunction

There are specific pelvic floor exercises which can help to deal with erectile dysfunction. However, recent research suggests that ordinary run of the mill exercise can also help. Just walking for half an hour, a few times a week can actually help with erectile dysfunction, because it boosts the circulation, and that's important, because to achieve and sustain an erection, you need good blood flow into the penis. Anything that helps the general circulation in the body will also help with that.

Here's the science bit. What helps the penis to become and remain erect is the health of the endothelium. That's the inner lining of the blood vessels, and it's a big aid to helping the blood flow smoothly and efficiently through the body. Regular exercise is known to maintain the health of the endothelium and thus keep the circulation at a healthy level. That means if you exercise regularly, not only will you keep your heart healthy, you could solve your erection problems at the same time.

There's good news here for the older guys too. Although erectile dysfunction can be a common problem of old age, regular exercise can hold back the aging process by counteracting the natural effects of aging on the blood vessels, and with it, the risk of problems in the bedroom in later life.

It doesn't have to mean pounding the streets or sweating it out in the gym either – walking and swimming are aerobic exercises which can help to keep the endothelium healthy and thus improve the circulation and enhance blood flow to the penis. Studies suggest that walking for 30 minutes a day can reduce the risk of developing erectile dysfunction by around 41%, so it's worth a try. It's also important to do something you enjoy in the way of exercise, because that way, you're more likely to stick with it. Almost said keep it up there, but maybe that's a pun too far!

Experts advise against cycling if you have potency problems, since it can cause damage to the nerves responsible for erections. However, it's okay to use an exercise cycle at home or in the gym, as the seat is likely to be wider and more comfortable than a conventional cycle saddle. Therefore, the risk of nerve damage is significantly reduced.

Exercise releases 'feel good' endorphins in the body, and that helps to combat stress and depression. Stress is very often a cause or a contributory factor in erectile dysfunction, and so is depression, and regular exercise can help tackle that. Also, if you need to lose a little weight and build muscle definition to give your self-esteem a boost, exercise can do that too. That's not to say that exercise is the answer to all your problems, but it can certainly help with them, and when you remember that exercise helps to lower blood pressure and stabilize blood glucose levels, you're taking a giant step towards good health, by preventing or treating hypertension and diabetes.

Another benefit of exercise is that it helps you to sleep well, so your body has time to do all the repairs it needs to do to keep you healthy. Lack of sleep can lead to fatigue during the day, and this can interfere with your ability to achieve and maintain an erection. And of course, lack of sleep can lead to stress and even heart disease, so as well as helping with your potency problems, exercise can also help you to stay generally healthy.

Exercise helps you to get slim and stay slim, and as well as improving your self-esteem and confidence, it could help you to avoid or overcome erectile dysfunction. Research suggests that a man with a 32" waist is 50% less likely to have problems with sexual performance than a man with a 42" waist, so there really is something in this exercise lark.

## Kegel Exercises

As has been mentioned before, there are certain pelvic floor exercises that men can do to help overcome erectile dysfunction. Also known as pelvic floor exercises, they are simple to perform, and can also help guard against other men's health problems such as urinary incontinence and prostate problems.

One really effective trick is to halt the flow of urine midstream several times. This identifies the muscles that need to be used in the Kegel exercises, because unless you identify and locate the right set of muscles, you won't gain any benefits from the exercises. To do the exercise, squeeze the muscles, hold the pose for a count of 5, then release. Repeat this 10 – 20 times, three times a day. The exercise can be done in any position, but it's a good idea to ring the changes and do them standing up, sitting down or lying down. That makes sure all the muscles are used.

Another good Kegel is to clench the muscles of the anus, as if you're trying to stop yourself from going to the toilet. Hold it for between 5 and 10 seconds, then release. Repeat 10 times. When you're doing Kegels, remember to keep breathing naturally. Don't hold your breath, because that will deprive the muscles of the oxygen they need to function properly. And just use the muscles you isolated and identified – resist the temptation to use muscles in your stomach, buttocks or thighs – that won't do you any favors at all.

Because these exercises strengthen the pelvic floor muscles and increase blood supply to the penis, they also have the potential to allow you to enjoy even better orgasms, since performing Kegels regularly enhances sexual sensation. This is partly because you become more in tune with your body as a result of isolating and working the pelvic floor muscles. That's a goal well worth striving for.

Exercise can help with erectile dysfunction in a number of ways. As well as helping you to lose weight and generally feel better about yourself, exercise improves blood flow all over the body, and particularly to the penis. It's also a great mood lifter, and can counteract any stress or depression you may be experiencing as a result of your condition. And if you perform specific pelvic floor exercises, as well as exercising generally, you'll increase your chances of enjoying a normal sex life once more.

Perhaps the best benefit of exercise is that, unlike Viagra, or other drugs which may be used to treat erectile dysfunction, it doesn't have any side effects, other than helping you to lose weight and feel fitter and healthier than ever before. If you don't exercise enough, maybe you should make an effort to be more active, for the sake of both your health and your sex life.

## Regular Cardio Vascular Exercises

Aside from increasing energy levels, improving muscle tone and reducing blood pressure, performing cardio vascular exercises on a regular basis can help reduce the risk for erectile dysfunction or if a man is already suffering from it, address it. Aside from allowing a man to achieve and maintain a healthy weight (remember obesity and its relationship to erectile dysfunction?), doing so can help a man get enough sleep, manage stress well, feel better about himself and improve heart health – all of which can help address erectile dysfunction issues. Such exercises include:

-Brisk walking;

-Dancing;

-Exercising on an elliptical trainer;

-Rowing;

-Running;

-Swimming; and

-Tae Bo.

To maximize the health benefits of regular cardio vascular exercising, the ideal duration and frequency is 20 to 30 minutes and 4 to 5 times per week, respectively. Don't overdo it nor take it too easy. If it's your first time to do cardio, consult with a doctor first to assess the optimal duration, intensity and frequency for you.

## Lifting Weights

One of the best ways to improve blood flow to the penis is to improving the health of blood vessels' inner lining called the endothelium. A healthy endothelium, according to prominent urology professor Dr. Wane Hellstrom, M.D., of the Tulane University School of Medicine, helps in improving a man's erections. Weight lifting or resistance training exercises can also help improve a man's endothelium health and consequently, blood flow to the penis.

In more ways than one, weight lifting can also help address psychological erectile dysfunction. How? Lifting weights makes a man physically stronger and look better (more muscular) ala Ryan Gosling or Ryan Reynolds. Looking better and being stronger can significantly improve a man's self-confidence and the way he sees himself as a sex object, both of which can stoke the fire of sexiness within and improve his ability to feel sexually aroused. And when a man is sexually aroused, you know what happens next.

## Push Ups

Since kegels have already been covered, and by now you have probably tried them six ways to Sunday, it is time for you to learn about other exercises that can help alleviate your erectile dysfunction.

When you think of the pushup you may not think that it is a particularly effective treatment for erectile dysfunction. After all, it is meant to exercise your upper body, such as your chest and shoulder muscles. How can pushups possibly help your erectile dysfunction, which has to do with a part of your body that is far removed from your upper body?

The first major way in which it helps is by improving blood circulation in your body. If you are suffering from poor circulation, it is important that you exercise in order to get your body into the practice of pumping blood to its various areas more efficiently.

Apart from this, pushups help greatly by strengthening your core. This includes the muscles of your abdomen as well as your lower back and, the most important muscles of all, your pelvic muscles. In order to stabilize yourself during pushups, you are going to have to strengthen your core muscles, which in turn means that your pelvic muscles are strengthened. This makes it a lot easier for you to get an erection, firstly because your pelvic muscles will become more powerful, and secondly because exercising your pelvic muscles is going to encourage blood flow to that particular part of your body. More blood flow means that it will be easier for you to get an erection.

Try to do about twenty to thirty pushups a day. You don't need to push yourself, just do enough that you get your blood pumping. Just remember to do them at least three and at most six time a week for the best results.

## The Plank

The plank is vastly different from the pushup, but it just as important at helping you overcome your erectile dysfunction. The plank essentially involves you face down, resting your upper body with your elbows and toes.

The way to do this is to get into position as if you were about to do a pushup and then descend until the length of your lower arm is what you are balancing your upper body with. Maintain this position for about a minute and then start doing pushups. You can use this as an interim between pushups in order to make your breather more intense. The more exercise you fill into a small space of time, the more effective your workout is going to be.

The benefit of the plank is that it targets your core just like pushups do. The difference is that with the plank you put a lot more focus on your groin and pelvic muscles. By mixing the plank up with pushups you are going to get your blood flowing and will then be essentially directing it to your pelvis which is going to make this workout super effective at alleviating your erectile dysfunction.

## Trampoline

A trampoline is tons of fun. It is a great way to bond with your kids, it's exhilarating, and it helps you slough off the stress of a long day and enjoy yourself. It also helps a great deal with erectile dysfunction. This is because trampoline jumping directs blood entirely to your lower body. One rather interesting fact about trampoline jumping is that the muscle that is used most while engaging in this activity is actually the pelvic muscle.

This makes trampoline jumping rather unique. It is one of the only exercises, apart from kegels, that puts emphasis on the pelvic muscles. An additional benefit of trampoline jumping is that it gets your blood flowing. While you are engaging in this activity, you are going to have a high pulse which means your blood is going to be flowing fast. Since the muscle that you are using the most right now is in your pelvis, a lot of this blood is going to end up flowing to your groin. This influx of blood is going to end up making it a lot easier for you to get an erection later on when you are trying to have sex.

## Yoga

Erectile dysfunction, especially psychological ones, are brought about by excess stress and fatigue.  One of the best ways to manage and control both is by fostering a very strong connection between body and mind, which can be done through exercises like yoga.

Yoga has been shown in many studies to be effective in terms of reducing stress and general tension of the body as well as in terms of improving one's breathing.  It's also generally helpful in improving a person's feeling of being well, which is also important for sexual arousal.

Yoga doesn't just help address psychological erectile dysfunction – it also helps address physiological ones.  It's because some forms of yoga exercises can help improve the pelvic region's blood circulation.  Since erections are primarily about blood flow in that region, it can help men's penises to "stand up and pay attention."

## Salsa

Let's face it, many people would like to have their cakes and eat them too by combining exercise and fun all in one session.  It's also worth noting that not everyone finds lifting weights and doing cardio to be fun.  The answer?  Try something like dancing – particularly salsa!

The beautiful thing about salsa dancing apart from being a good cardiovascular exercise is that it's something that a couple can enjoy together. Not only does it burn much calories, it can also be so much fun with the music and the opportunity to develop more intimacy between both partners, which can translate to a much better sexual relationship. Improved blood flow and emotional well being – what more can you ask for in an exercise, eh?

## Essential Oils For Erectile Dysfunction

Physical and psychological factors can also influence erectile dysfunction. Essential oils can help reduce impotence by stimulating blood flow and taking care of any underlying psychological issues you're experiencing.

Essential oils have already been useful for ages to cure many health problems and impotence isn't an exception.

Below are some essential oils which will help cure erectile dysfunction.

- **Basil:** The smell of basil arouses sexual instincts. Additionally, it calms down stress.
- **Black Pepper:** It relieves exhaustion and melts self-doubt. It restores sexual energy by warming the human body and alleviating emotions.
- **Cardamom:** Due to its aphrodisiac properties, cardamom is employed to boost sexual desire and

libido. It contains cineole, a substance that influences the central nervous system.

- **Cedarwood:** This oil arouses sensual feelings and improves sexual response. It also calms concerns and fears regarding sex.
- **Clary Sage:** This herb supports greater sleep, reduces anxiety, and relieves depression. It also increases sexual interest and arouses sexual thoughts. It is best employed for impotence caused by mental elements because it opens negative feelings and removes inhibitions.
- **Ginger:** It is an aphrodisiac. It stimulates sexual desires and warms the human body, thus, increasing libido.
- **Geranium:** It relaxes the muscles and helps relieve stress, fatigue, and anxiety. It is also an aphrodisiac, antidepressant, and antioxidant.
- **Jasmine:** Its nice, floral scent is very intoxicating and relaxing. It's also an aphrodisiac. It warms your body and promotes deep sleep. Also, it burns up anger and disappointment.
- **Juniper:** This essential oil is better for ED on account of emotional and mental elements. It removes relationship insecurities, arouses love and sex, and promotes self-confidence.
- **Lavender:** Its flowery, intoxicating, sweet scent arouses sexual emotions. In a report about male reaction to aromatherapy, lavender is demonstrated to increase penile blood flow by 40%. Additionally, it wards off stress and anxiety.
- **Neroli:** This oil can be an aphrodisiac, and it effectively releases anxiety regarding sex.

- **Rose:** It increases intimacy in couples. It also advances the sensation of love and dispels fear of intimacy.
- **Sandalwood:** It stimulates delicate emotions and refreshes the mind and body. It's also an aphrodisiac and assists with frigidity and impotence.
- **Vetiver:** This oil reduces concerns and tensions. It is sexually stimulating and strengthens sexual desires.
- **Ylang-ylang:** It's used as an aphrodisiac. It revitalizes overall power, relaxes the body, and encourages soothing sleep. It also relieves depression and stress.

You can add these essential oils to your bath water or rub them into your genitals. Be sure you combine them with a carrier oil before using as a massage oil or immediately using on your skin.

Listed here are essential oil mixtures for treating erectile dysfunction.

**Blend 1**

20 drops basil

15 drops clary sage

10 drops ylang-ylang

1 drop clove

1 drop patchouli

1 oz. jojoba oil or coconut oil

Combine all oils in a glass bottle. You may use it directly on your genitals and massage some on your pelvic area. You can even add this mixture to your bath.

## Blend 2

30 drops clary sage

30 drops fennel

20 drops sage

10 drops yarrow

5 drops peppermint

Mix oils carefully. To use directly on your skin, add 1 oz. jojoba oil, sesame seed oil, or coconut oil. You can even use this mix in your diffuser, preferably one hour or 3 minutes before having sex. You can also add this mix to your warm bath. Mix oils in 1 tbsp. honey and mix in your warm bathwater.

## Blend 3

30 drops geranium

30 drops rosewood

15 drops ylang-ylang

10 drops myrrh

10 drops black pepper

Combine the oils in 1 oz. jojoba oil and use it to massage your top, back, and pelvic area. You can even use it on your genitals. You may also include this blend in your warm bath.

**Blend 4**

10 drops rosewood

1 drop sandalwood

8 drops clary sage

6 drops thyme

6 drops ylang-ylang

**4 drops coriander**

Mix all oils and add to your diffuser or light. Use about an hour before bedtime. You may also add this combination to your bath. Utilize it in the morning and the evening for maximum benefits.

Some people have extremely sensitive skin. Before you use any of these mixes directly on your skin, be sure to do a skin patch test. Apply a small amount of your chosen mix on your hand and dab it at the trunk of your palm. Wait for one hour and look for any responses. If you have none, you can use the blend safely for your diffuser, shower, or topical use.

## Herbs for the Treatment Of Erectile Dysfunction

The needed herbs for the treatment of erectile dysfunctions include:

1. Maca root
2. Gingko Biloba
3. Irish Sea Moss
4. Panax Ginseng
5. Yohimbe

## Maca Root

Maca root is a very effective herbal medicine that has been used by the Peruvians for over 3,000 years. This herb is very rich with some compound and nutrients like: vitamins-B, fatty acids, amino acids, phytonutrients, zinc, calcium, selenium, magnesium and iron.

Till date this herb is very effective for the improvement of fertility (increase sperm count and semen) for men, enhance sexual urge (libido), treatment of erectile dysfunctions that is caused by antidepressants, anemia (tired blood), reliefs anxiety and depression, improve energy and stamina level, relief symptoms of menopause, boost the immune system etc.

**Precaution And Side Effects Of Consuming Maca Root?**

Till at the time of written this book, Maca root is 100% safe for men to consume except for women that it has some side effect which I am not going to talk about since this book is completely design for men.

**Maca Root Dosage**

The dosage for Maca root depends on what you are using it to treat. However, the various dosages include:

1. FOR INFERTILITY: to improve your fertility by increasing your semen and sperm count, take Maca root twice pay day for 4 month
2. FOR BOOSTING OF LIBIDO AND TREATMENT OF ERECTILE DYSFUNCTION: to enhance your libido and erection, take Maca root twice per day for 12days.
3. FOR ANXIETY AND DEPRESSION: to relief anxiety and depression, take Maca root twice per day for 10days
4. FOR BOOSTING OF IMMUNE SYSTEM, ENERGY AND STAMINA LEVEL AND TO RELIEF THE SYMPTOMS OF MANOPAUSE: take Maca root, twice per day for 2weeks

**The Preparation of Maca Root**

To prepare Maca root, kindly take the steps below:

1. Harvest some Maca root, wash it and dry it. Once it is dry, pound or chops it into smaller pieces.

2. Measure1teaspoon and pour it into your ceramic pot with 8ounce of water and boil it for 10-15 minute.
3. Step it down and strain it.

Alternatively, measure 1tablespoon of Maca root powder if you buy it online and add it to any of your choice smoothie or juice twice per day.

## Ginkgo Biloba

Ginkgo Biloba is an herbal plant that has been used by the Chinese for more than 200 million years ago. This herb is very effective for the treatment of most of the physiological causes of erectile dysfunctions. However, because of the compound and nutrients that Ginkgo Biloba contains, research has it that tea made with the leaves of this herb is very potent in treating of anxiety, Alzheimer disease (dementia), stroke, high blood pressure, depression, multiple sclerosis etc. Don't forget that all these diseases are causes of erectile dysfunctions and this herb will help to eliminate erectile dysfunctions from it root-caused.

### Precaution and Side Effects of Consuming Ginkgo Biloba

Tea made with the leaves of Ginkgo Biloba is likely safe but if it is taken in excess (overdose), you might suffer from minor side effects like: dizziness, forceful heartbeat, stomach upset and headache.

## Ginkgo Biloba Dosage

The dosage for Ginkgo Biloba depends on what you are using it to treat. However, the various dosages include:

1. For the treatment of depression, anxiety, high blood pressure and blood clot, take ginkgo biloba three times per day for 4 weeks (1 month)
2. For stroke, take ginkgo biloba, 3times daily for 14-30days
3. For Alzheimer disease (dementia) and multiple sclerosis take ginkgo biloba three times per day for 12month.

## The Preparation of Ginkgo Biloba:

For the preparation of Ginkgo Biloba, you will need to harvest some fresh leaves of Ginkgo Biloba, wash it and dry it. Once it is dried, chop it into smaller pieces and follow the under-listed steps:

1. Boil 8ounce of water and turn off the fire and measure 2teaspoon of the chopped or pounded leaves and pour it into the boiled water.
2. Allow it to steam for 5-10 minutes and strain it using a strainer or filter.
3. You are done.

## Irish Sea Moss

Irish Sea Moss is also known as Sea Moss. It is a red alga that people have used it long before now for food but today it is used for the treatment of various health disorders. Because of how rich this herb is with over 92 minerals that the human body needs out of the 102, I strongly recommend this herb for the treatment of erectile dysfunctions, calming and boosting of the immune system, enrich overall mood, speed up healing, boost energy and stamina level and also, reliefs; arthritis, pain and swelling of the joint cause by inflammation, combat different types of infections etc.

## The Precaution and Side Effects Of Consuming Irish Sea Moss

Irish Sea Moss is likely safe if consume in an average dosage but if consume in overdose, there is tendency of some mild side effects like

1. Burning sensation or itching of the mouth
2. Spew out or vomiting
3. Stomach upset or irritation
4. Nausea.

## The Dosage Of Irish Sea Moss

The dosage of Irish Sea Moss is generic. All you have to do is to consume Irish Seas moss once per day for 2 weeks upward. (Preferably in the morning)

## Preparation of Irish Sea Moss

To prepare Irish Sea Moss tea, take the under-listed steps:

1. Get either the gel or powdery form of Irish Sea Moss.
2. Boil 8ounce of water in a ceramic pot and turn the water into your tea cup/mug
3. Pour into the boiled water, 1 tablespoon of Irish Sea Moss gel or the powdery form depending on the one you have.
4. Cover the tea cup/mug and allow it to steep for 10-15minutes to dissolve completely.
5. You are done. You can now enjoy your warm tea made with Irish Sea Moss.

## Panax Ginseng

Panax Ginseng is an herbal plant from northeastern China, Siberia and Korea. I included this herb because of its potency to treat physiological causes of erectile dysfunctions such as; boosting of the brain functionality, treatment of multiple sclerosis, Alzheimer's disease, heart failure, diabetes, high blood pressure etc. This herb is also very effective for the treatment of erectile dysfunctions such as; boosting of libido by increasing response to sexual stimuli, prevent premature ejaculation (early orgasm), enhance athletic performance and boost energy and stamina level and a lot more.

## The Precautions and Side Effects of Consuming Panax Ginseng

This herb is likely safe when consumed for the period of 6 month. Anything more than 6 months, can lead to some side effect like:

1. Insomnia,
2. Increase heart rate
3. Loss of appetite
4. Low/high blood pressure
5. Itching
6. Mood swing etc.

Therefore, this herb should not be used for more than 4month.

## Dosage of Panax Ginseng

FOR THE PREVENTION OF PREMATURE EJACULATION, HEART FAILURE, DIABETES, take this herb 3times daily for 16weeks.

FOR ALZHEIMER DISEASE (DEMENTIA) AND MULTIPLE SCLEROSIS, take Panax Ginseng 3 times daily for 12weeks

FOR HIPERTENSION, ANXIETY AND BOOSTING OF LIBIDO, take Panax Ginseng 3times per day for 8weeks

## The Preparation of Panax Ginseng

Harvest some fresh root of Panax Ginseng, wash it and dried it. Pound it or chop it into smaller pieces and the steps below:

1. Measure 8-10 ounce of water and pour it into your ceramic pot and measure 2teaspoon of the chopped Panax Ginseng and add it to the water.
2. Boil the mixture for 15 minutes. Once it is boiled, step it down for 5 minutes and strain it using a strainer.

## Yohimbe

Yohimbe is an evergreen herbal tree in which tea made with the bark of this herbal evergreen tree contains yohimbine chemicals that helps to counteract the side effects of almost all depression medication. That's not all as it also helps to boost sexual urge, treat and prevent sexual problems, obesity, high blood pressure, enrich mood, relief anxiety and depression, boost energy and stamina level and a lot more.

**The Precautions and Side Effects of Consuming Yohimbe**

If you consume yohimbe in a moderate amount or as tea, its side effect is almost impossible for a short period of time but if you consume it for a very long period of time (6month) and above in high dose, there are some severe side effects like:

1. Heart attack or rapid heartbeat
2. Seizure and
3. Kidney failure.

However, it has some minor side effect which includes:

1. Stomach irritation
2. Excitation
3. Anxiety
4. Tremor
5. Dizziness
6. High blood pressure
7. Sleep problems
8. Sinus pain
9. Headache
10. Drooling
11. Nausea
12. Vomiting
13. Frequent urination
14. Irritability and
15. Rash.

However, to prevent and avoid all the above side effects, only use the tea of this herb and don't use it for more than 3 months.

**The Dosage of Yohimbe**

FOR BOOSTING OF LIBIDO, ENEGY AND STAMINA LEVEL, take Yohimbe 3 times per day for 21days

FOR DEPRESSION, ANXIETY AND MOOD SWING, take Yohimbe 3 times per day for 10days.

FOR SEXUAL PROBLEMS, OBESITY, HIGH BLOOD PRESSURE, take Yohimbe 3 times per day for 4weeks.

**The Preparation Of Yohimbe**

Harvest some barks of Yohimbe, chops or pound it into smaller pieces and dry it or you can make an order online. Once you have it, you can take the steps below:

1. Measure 8ounce of water and 1-1½ teaspoon of the chopped or pounded Yohimbe and pour it into your ceramic pot and boil it for 10-15minute.
2. Step it down and strain it using a strainer or filter.

## *Diet Type Options To Overcome Erectile Dysfunction*

Diet has been reiterated time and time again as a solution for erectile dysfunction, but it can be tough to solve the problem if the only advice you're going to get is to 'eat healthily.' That being mentioned, this section is devoted to adhering to unique diet programs that can help in the treatment of erectile dysfunction exacerbated by diabetes, elevated blood pressure, and heart problems.

## DASH (Dietary Approaches to Stop Hypertension) DIET

The DASH (Dietary Approaches to Stop Hypertension) Diet is highly advised for those with high blood pressure. If you suffer from hypertension, this is the perfect food regimen to lower your blood pressure and hopefully reduce the instances of erectile dysfunction.

## What Is It?

The DASH Diet focuses on getting sufficient amounts of nutrients while paying heed to portion control. Doctors often recommend it due to its comprehensive approach. It can be quite easy to follow because the diet doesn't just prescribe what food items to eat but also establishes a daily limit, therefore giving you a clear view of what can and cannot be done.

### *General Principles*

Here's what you should know about the DASH Diet:

- There are two versions of the DASH Diet: the Standard Sodium and the Low Sodium. The first one limits your sodium intake to just 2,300 mg per day, while the other one lowers it to just 1,500 per day. For the sake of comparison, a regular diet contains 3,500 mg sodium per day.
- An additional limit is 2,000 calories each day. Hence – the DASH Diet requires you to eat no more than 2,000 calories each day, the sodium content of which must NOT exceed 2,300mg.

### *Vegetable Servings*

Vegetables should be treated as a main dish rather than a side dish. Under the DASH Diet, you should consume at least four servings of a variety of vegetables daily. Try to measure each serving per cup, which means you can eat as much as 1 cup of vegetables during breakfast. Leafy green vegetables are the best kind when it comes to high blood pressure. Note that fresh and frozen vegetables are the best options, while canned vegetables should only be bought if the first two are not available. Always choose the 'low sodium' canned goods.

## Dairy Servings

This includes all milk derivatives rich in vitamin D, calcium, and even protein. Now, not all dairy products are DASH Diet approved. It's important to opt for the ones that are low in fat if not completely fat-free. Two to three dairy servings every day are acceptable and should keep you well provided in terms of calcium. Those that are lactose intolerant should try a lactase medicine that is available over the counter – this will help you digest lactose better. Yogurt is by far the most flexible source of dairy today and should keep you happy with the choices, especially since you can boost the flavor by adding fruit into the mix.

## Nuts and Seed Servings

Since nuts and seeds are rich in calories, they should be eaten in moderation – at least 4 to 5 servings per week. They contain high amounts of potassium and magnesium, which can help against certain cancers even while lowering instances of high blood pressure. Don't be concerned about the high-fat content of nuts – this is good fat and will help fight hypertension.

Nuts can be consumed as crunchy snacks, or you can opt to add them to your salad, putting a whole new dimension to leafy green as you feel a satisfying crunch with each bite.

## Fruit Servings

The DASH Diet is ideal for those with hypertension and NOT with diabetes because it recommends up to 5 servings of fruit each day. Despite the health attributes of fruit, the fact is that it contains sufficient amounts of sugar that could prove negative for a diabetic.

Fruits are wonderfully flexible in that they contain all sorts of vitamins and minerals, depending on which fruit you favor. Avoid avocado and coconuts since they tend to be high in fat, but otherwise, the fruit world is your oyster!

You may incorporate the fruit into your regular yogurt servings or just enjoy it as a treat or snack. Canned fruit and frozen fruit work too, but nothing beats fresh servings. If you're going to buy something canned, make sure it has zero or low sodium.

## Meat and Fish Servings

Yes – you can eat meat on a DASH Diet, provided that they're lean rather than the fatty kind that comes cheap. This can be consumed with a max of 6 portions or fewer every day. Please note that meat and fish are interchangeable, but you should NOT eat meat alone. Fish is crucial because it supplies your body with much-needed omega-3 fatty acids, which is beneficial for practically all types of health issues.

### Sweet Items

Sweets are also not entirely banned from the DASH Diet – but it makes sense to limit their serving to just five a week or less if you can manage it. The 'sweets' should also be limited to sorbet, jelly, jam, low-fat cookies, fruit juices, hard candy, etc. You can choose artificial sweeteners but don't rely on them too much. Remember: sugar has no added value, so it's mainly consumed to satisfy your sweet tooth.

### Fat and Oil Servings

As mentioned, avocado is one fruit that's high in the good kind of fat, so if you want to kill two birds with one stone, this is the type to go for. Keep your fat consumption to just 2 to 3 servings every day because too much fat can lead to heart problems. Ideally, you should focus only on monounsaturated fat and avoiding large amounts of cheese, margarine, cream, eggs, and anything fried.

Everything else not mentioned in the diet should be consumed in moderation or not, including alcohol and caffeine. Note that there are instances when the food items overlap – for example, avocado contains fat which means that in some instances, they can be counted as fruits and fat – thereby allowing you to cross off TWO DASH Diet requirements in one sitting. Be mindful of these overlaps to make sure you're getting the amount you need. Check your blood pressure weekly or even daily to see if the DASH Diet is working for you. Erectile Dysfunction symptoms should decrease pursuant to better health.

## Mediterranean Diet

The Mediterranean Diet (MD) is perhaps one of the most praised diets today, ranking among those best used for heart health and weight loss purposes.

### What Is It?

The diet is named such because it follows the diet of people in the Mediterranean. Research shows that those who live in the Mediterranean and follow this particular system in their food regimen have lower instances of cardiovascular problems – hence the sudden interest in bringing MD to the shores of the United States. Additional perks of this diet include reduced risks of Alzheimer's, cancer, and Parkinson's.

### *General Principles*

The best thing about this diet is that it does not force you to count calories. The General Principle is quite simple: eat as if you live in one of the countries bordering the Mediterranean, such as Greece. The diet proceeds by viewing food options as a pyramid divided into four key categories. Here's a rundown of each of them.

### *Primary Level – Fruits, Vegetables, Grains, Oils, Herbs, Etc.*

This is the Mediterranean Diet's first and most critical standard. The focus is vegetables, fruits, and grain in that particular order. Your main fare would be leady greens with fruit as the primary source of sugar. Bread is an important part of daily consumption, but it's usually whole wheat which is healthier compared to the white version, plus the fact that Greeks often skip butter and margarine – preferring their bread toasted with none of the garnishing often added in the American version. As for rice, the option is usually brown.

The importance of olive oil in the diet is also astounding, as it can be used in almost every recipe. With olive oil containing high amounts of omega-3 essential fatty acids, the addition of this further lowers heart risk issues.

### Secondary Level – Fish and Seafood

The second most prevalent addition to MD is fish and other types of seafood. Fish is another good source of omega-3 fatty acids while at the same time containing vitamins, minerals, and protein necessary to keep the body well-supplied and healthy. Options such as tuna, salmon, and mackerel are perhaps the most prevalent in this particular diet.

### Third Level – Poultry, Cheese, Eggs, Etc.

Dairy products, eggs, and poultry occupy the third level and should be eaten sparingly – no more than twice to three days a week in limited amounts. Keep in mind that although poultry is technically meat, it is only derived from chicken or turkey and NOT beef, pork, etc. If you're going to consume dairy, make sure you're getting the low-fat or zero-fat versions.

## Meat and Sweets

Occupying the topmost portion are meats and sweets, which, in this case, make them UNDESIRABLE for those following the Mediterranean Diet. Of course, that doesn't mean that you should ban them altogether from your diet, but it stands to reason that their consumption should be limited to only the smallest amount. Once or twice a month in reasonable proportions should be enough – especially when it comes to sweets. Meat must also be lean – the fatty portion removed to make sure that it doesn't affect your cholesterol levels.

## What Else?

The primary goal of the Mediterranean Diet is to make sure you only get the good kind of fat derived from fruits and vegetables. Hence, anything processed is often shunned in favor of fresh versions of food. Other considerations under this food regimen are:

- Red wine is permitted but must be limited to just one glass per day. Any other kind of alcohol is best avoided.
- Salt and sugar as seasoning is also forbidden. Greeks tend to use herbs and spices for their food which includes thyme, basil, parsley, pepper, and others
- As mentioned, olive oil is heavily used in MD with butter and regular oil limited if not completely removed from the regimen.

The Mediterranean Diet is amazing that it has gained so much popularity that there are now cookbooks focused solely on this discipline. Hence, you'll find that MD won't be as restrictive as the pyramid suggests. A few months into this particular diet and you should be able to reverse the negative effects of cardiovascular issues, including those of erectile dysfunction.

## Glycemic Index

The Glycemic Index is not a diet per se but rather a guideline that helps diabetics figure out whether certain food types are compatible with their nutritional needs. If you suffer from erectile dysfunction with diabetes as the primary culprit, this particular diet will follow.

### What Is It?

Also known as GI, the Glycemic Index is essentially a ranking system based on the ability of certain foods to raise glucose levels in the blood. The food items are ranked 0 to 100, with the low-GI food items generally considered the best for those suffering from diabetes. The system focuses on carbohydrate content and how long it takes to convert into glucose or sugar.

Food with a fast conversion rate naturally spikes up sugar in the blood, while those with a low conversion rate provide a slow and steady flow of energy. This is why the GI Diet is also used by those who want to lose weight.

There are three categories to GI:

- High GI – 70 and higher
- Medium GI – 56 to 69
- Low GI – 1 to 55

You should be eating food items that are within that Low GI level with moderate amounts of Medium GI and essentially nothing of those in the High GI bracket. The question is: how do you know the GI level of the current food you're eating? The internet answers that one thing with databases is letting you enter specific food items and find out exactly where they rank in the index.

*Low GI*

Low GI food items generally include vegetables and whole grains. Oatmeal and bran breakfast cereals are also included in the list, as well as various fleshy fruit items.

*Medium GI*

Some fruits fall under the Medium GI classification, including banana, pineapple, raisins, and sweet corn. Breakfast cereals can also fall under this category, depending on their specific makeup. In truth, the lines between Low and Medium GI can be somewhat blurred, hence, the need to check and make sure which one you're getting.

*High GI*

High GI includes a lot of sweet items, including ice cream, hard candy, and white bread. White rice and potatoes are also included in the list. Packaged food items are generally high on the GI list and should therefore be avoided as much as possible.

**Some Considerations**

The main issue with the GI Diet is that it doesn't take into account portion control. It is to be understood that you will be the one exercising control over the amount of food you're eating. As a general rule, whenever you're consuming anything with a high GI, consume as little of it as possible. However, with Low GI food, you can eat as many as you want without worrying about the results too much.

*Vitamins*

Aside from having the proper diet and taking herbal supplements, vitamin supplements can also prevent and treat erectile dysfunction. Below are the essential vitamins needed to improve your erections:

**Vitamin A** - this is a very important vitamin in terms of regulating progesterone. Progesterone is the most essential progestogen hormone of the human body. One of its many functions is stimulating the sexual drive of an individual (both male and female). And for a male person, it can help in treating erectile problems.

Foods rich in Vitamin A: green, leafy vegetables, yellow fruits, squash, fish, milk.

**Vitamin B** - most of the complex B vitamins are able to give positive effects when it comes to penile erection. Vitamin B1, or thiamin, strengthens nerves and vascular organs that helps improve penile functions. It also provides more energy all throughout the day which can translate into more energy during sexual intercourse as well. Vitamin B3, or niacin, stimulates the body's systems to produce more sex hormones and improves the cardiovascular system as well.

Meanwhile, vitamin B9, or folic acid, helps increase sperm count and potency, which leads to more lengthy erections. Vitamin B12, or cobalamin, is another vitamin that strengthens the nerves and blood cells of the body.

Foods rich in Vitamin B: pork, liver, carrots, oatmeal (B1); mushrooms, eggs, (B3); pasta, bread, cereals (B9); and meat and other animal dairy products like milk and cheese (B12).

**Vitamin C** - apart from helping your body create more sex hormones and boosting your sperm count, vitamin C also strengthens your vascular nerves, arteries, veins, and capillaries for better blood flow. An added benefit is that it helps lower bad cholesterol and increase stored energy, which will not only make your erection last longer during intercourse, but your performance as well.

Foods rich in Vitamin C: citrus fruits, tomatoes, guava, cabbage, chili peppers, red bell pepper, green bell pepper, cauliflower.

**Vitamin D** - a recent study at the University of Milan in Italy regarding sexual disorders reported that insufficient supply of vitamin D in the body can lead to an erectile dysfunction. The study revealed that all of the men that had erection problems have 20% lesser amounts of vitamin D in their systems as compared to those who have natural erections. They have also found out that vitamin D is responsible in maximizing the use of nitric oxide in the body. And nitric oxide stimulates the vascular muscles to relax, making them more open so blood can flow efficiently. And you know that when blood is flowing freely and efficiently, erections are more intense as well.

Foods rich in Vitamin D: Mushrooms, liver, fish, egg yolks, cheese.

**Vitamin E** - this vitamin is a powerful antioxidant, which, like vitamin D, helps stimulate the circulation of nitric oxide in the body. Aside from helping your body fight cancer cells from multiplying and decreasing your risk of having heart attacks, vitamin E can help you with your penile issues as well. It also stimulates the production of prostaglandins, which are powerful hormones that increase libido.

Foods rich in Vitamin E include: almonds, raw seeds, hazelnuts, kale, spinach.

**Other nutrients that help improve erectile problems:**

**Zinc** - as already mentioned above, zinc improves the potency of sperm cells, and it increases testosterone and libido levels too. A 250 mg supplement a day can help you a lot if you have erection problems.

Foods rich in zinc include: oysters, shellfish, nuts, chicken, salmon, lamb, beef, and turkey.

**Omega-3 fatty acids** - a healthier and stronger heart leads to a more productive sex life and penile erection as well. And omega-3 fatty acids helps a lot with regards to preserving your heart. It also increases the generation of nitric oxide in the body.

Foods rich in omega-3 fatty acids include: salmon, tuna, vegetable oils, soybean, flaxseeds, kale, spinach.

**Selenium** - around half of selenium in a man's body is found in his testicles and semen canals. If he is suffering from selenium insufficiency, then chances are that he will suffer from erectile dysfunction as well.

Foods rich in selenium include: brown rice, chia seeds, Brazil nuts, shitake mushrooms, broccoli, spinach.

**Magnesium** - this trace mineral is responsible for producing estrogen, androgen, and brain chemicals that is responsible for boosting libido levels. If you are low on this, then it will be difficult for your penis to have an erection.

Foods rich in magnesium include: leafy vegetables, avocado, fish, beans, whole grains, nuts, seeds, bananas, dark chocolate.

## List of Best Foods for Erectile Dysfunction

While there is no miracle food that can help prevent or treat erectile dysfunction, the good news is that, there is evidence that some types of food may help.

According to urology experts, the sheer potency of certain kinds of food in treating erectile dysfunction lies in the health dilemma's vascular origins. Erectile dysfunction is almost always caused by poor blood supply to the penis; hence, food that can promote the proper functioning of the vascular system may also help in the treatment and prevention of erectile dysfunction.

Below are some of the best foods that may help in the prevention and treatment of erection problems:

### 1. Beets and Green Leafy Vegetables

Green leafy vegetables, such as spinach and celery, may help increase blood circulation since they contain loads of nitrates. Beet juice is also found to be highly concentrated with nitrates. Nitrates are highly touted as effective vasodilators, which means that they are capable of opening up the blood vessels and hence promote better blood flow. In 1998, the United States

Food and Drug Administration or US-FDA approved the very first medication for erectile dysfunction. Thereafter, several case reports which cited the positive impacts of nitrates for erectile dysfunction have been publicized. Most medications for erectile dysfunction are based on the relaxing properties of nitrates on the blood vessels which deliver blood to the penis.

**2. Dark Chocolate**

In a recent study published in the journal "Circulation", it has been revealed that dark chocolate contains flavonoids which can help boost circulation. This could be beneficial for those with erection problems caused by poor blood circulation. Flavonoids contain antioxidant properties that safeguard plants from toxic materials and aid in repairing cell damage. According to recent studies, flavonoids, as well as other types of antioxidants have similar impacts on people. They aid in reducing cholesterol and lowering blood pressure, both of which are crucial factors that contribute to erection problems.

**3. Pistachio**

It has recently been reported that men suffering from erectile dysfunction showed considerable improvements in their sexual issues upon eating pistachio nuts on a daily basis. The positive effects of pistachio on sexual problems may be attributed to arginine, a type of protein which helps relax the blood vessels that supply blood to the penis. This is one perfect example of how proper blood circulation is good for sexual health.

## 4. Oyster

Oyster has been touted as an excellent aphrodisiac since time immemorial; one reason behind this is that oysters contain high amounts of zinc, which significantly contributes to the production of testosterone (a male hormone). Low levels of this male hormone are known to be one of the causes of erectile dysfunction. On the other hand, a study presented at a meeting of the American Chemical Society, suggested that raw shellfish may contain substances that can promote the release of sexual hormones in women and men alike.

## 5. Watermelon

Certain studies suggest that watermelon has effects similar to those of Viagra, a popular erectile dysfunction drug, and may also help boost overall sexual desire. Watermelon is packed with potent ingredients called phytonutrients which have amazing antioxidant properties. One of the benefits of phytonutrients is that they help relax the blood vessels which deliver blood to the penis. While watermelon is composed mostly of water, it also contains components which may work wonders for your sexual enjoyment and for your heart.

## 6. Grapefruit and Tomatoes

Lycopene is among the best phytonutrients when it comes to boosting sexual desire and promoting blood circulation. Lycopene is abundant in deep-red fruits, including grapefruit and tomato. According to some studies, lycopene may be best absorbed when combined with oily vegetables such as spinach and avocados. So, you may want to try making your own erectile dysfunction-combatting salad. In addition to this, some studies show that antioxidant compounds, such as lycopene, can help combat prostate cancer and infertility.

The bottom line: Your best bet to avoid and cure erection problems is to follow a diet that is good for your circulation and your heart. Other foods that can help bring better blood circulation include red wine, tea, onions, peanuts, apples and cranberries. If you properly care for your vascular health, you will have a higher chance of avoiding the most common causes of erection problems.

## Other Tips for Treating Erectile Dysfunction

In addition to the different home remedies for erectile dysfunction, we can change certain habits in our life that could influence when it comes to suffering from sexual impotence.

## Consume (a lot) Olive Oil

Increase the consumption of liquid gold, fruits, vegetables, pasta and everything that includes the applauded Mediterranean diet. It is good to the heart, and many cases of ED, in which impotence is a symptom rather than a condition, are caused by cardiovascular issues. 80% of erectile dysfunction cases are caused by vascular problems. Maintaining a healthy blood pressure and cholesterol level will enhance your sexual activity. The testosterone in the fat will be transformed into female hormones, and cholesterol will reduce the blood flow to the penis.

## Get Around (but not by bike)

If you suffer from erection problems, don't lie on the couch. Sport will improve your blood circulation and therefore your performance. With exercise, we are going to get our vascular tree ready to carry blood to all organs, including the penis. Any discipline is good, except cycling. The perineum is traumatized, and the arteries that transport blood to the penis are injured as a result of the saddles. They even create that sensation of numbness in the glans that some cyclists have.

## Give the Herbs a Chance

Arginine is an amino acid that helps with sexual intercourse by increasing blood flow. Arginine is found in protein-rich foods like soybeans, brown rice, chicken, nuts, and dairy, and of course, in a bunch of herbal medicine bottles. Taking two to five grams of arginine before bedtime or an hour before sexual activity is good for the body. Some plants have aphrodisiac powers, they increase libido and potency

## Relax and Meditate

Another great way to treat erectile dysfunction naturally is to do relaxation exercises. Some disciplines such as yoga or breathing exercises are excellent to ward off stress. So, we finish as we started, avoid stress and accustom your body to good lifestyle habits, it will thank you!

Stress is responsible for many health disorders, including ED. And not only that, impotence can generate stress for those who suffer from it, so it is a vicious cycle. Stress causes the release of adrenaline, which constricts the arteries leading to the penis; no one can get an erection when they are stressed.

Try to get away from anxiety: relax, regularly practice breathing exercises, try to disconnect from work and relativize problems. You will see how your spirits will be lifted.

## Make a Lot of Love

One study showed that the most sexually active men had a higher incidence of erectile dysfunction than those who had less sex.

It is clear that this is a preventive measure: if you can't do it, how the hell will you repeat? However, scientists from the University Hospital of Tampere (Finland) showed in 2008 that men who have sex more frequently are less likely to suffer from this problem. In other words, the more sex you have, the less likely you are to have erectile dysfunction. Going into detail, they discovered that the problem had an incidence of 7.9% in men who had sex less than once a week, 3.2% in those who did it once a week and 1.6% among those athletes who practiced it three or more times every seven days.

Ultimately, it is about taking care of your lifestyle, as a study by the University of Adelaide (Australia) lit up last year, which with this surprising headline drew powerfully attention: *Erectile dysfunction can be cured without medication.* What the experts proposed was not so difficult to fulfill (or yes, depending on how you look at it): improve your weight and take care of nutrition, do more sports, drink less alcohol, sleep better at night and identify risk factors such as diabetes, hypertension or cholesterol. 29% of the men analyzed managed, with healthier habits, to overcome impotence.

**Take Away Stress**

Another common cause of impotence is stress. When a person suffers from erectile dysfunction, stress is often increased, so they enter a vicious cycle in which stress fuels impotence, and this condition increases stress. The adrenaline that a man experiences during periods of stress closes the arteries responsible for transporting blood to the penis, so it is not possible for an erection to occur.

## Stop Smoking

Men who smoke are at higher risk of being affected by ED, and the more cigarettes they smoke, the greater the risk. This is supported by a 2007 study from Tulane University (Louisiana, USA). The analysis, based on an examination of more than 7,000 men in China between 2000 and 2001, added that 22.7% of cases of dysfunction in that country were attributable to tobacco use.

Tobacco is another risk factor that can lead to impotence. Therefore, men who smoke are at greater risk of suffering from this sexual problem.

## Keep your Body Active

A sedentary lifestyle does not help when it comes to improving impotence. On the contrary, if we decide to get up from the sofa and do a little exercise, such as going for a run or walking, we improve blood circulation.

# Chapter Six: Enjoying Sex In Spite of Erectile Dysfunction

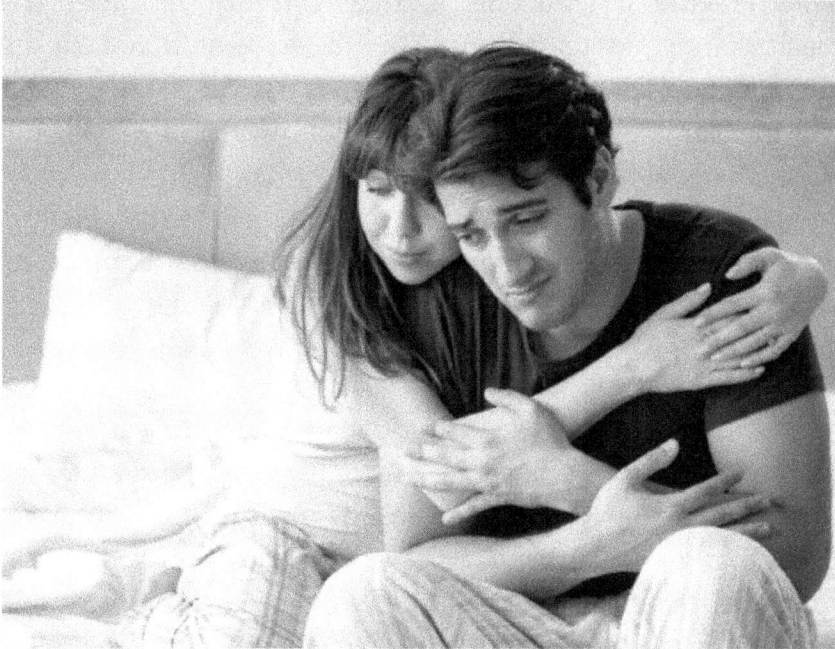

Just because you have erectile dysfunction doesn't mean you can't enjoy sex. There are a lot of people out there who enjoy full and happy sex lives despite the fact that they suffer from erectile dysfunction. In fact, there are a lot of people that can go their entire lives suffering from erectile dysfunction and not have any major problems with their sex lives. There are a number of activities you and your partner can do in order to enjoy sex and intimacy together that won't put pressure on you to get erect.

## Mutual Masturbation

One of the biggest reasons that you might be suffering from erectile dysfunction is that you are too used to masturbating on your own. The vagina would not be an adequate tool for getting you erect because you just don't find it as pleasurable as the firm grip of your own hand. When you masturbate, you tend to know exactly what to do in order to have a pleasurable experience. It's your body after all. Hence, the orgasms you feel when you masturbate would appear to be a lot more intense than the one's you'd be feeling with your partner.

However, this does not mean that you cannot be intimate with your partner and masturbate at the same time. Masturbation is a great way to enjoy each other's bodies. Usually when you masturbate you probably think of someone, a fantasy or something similar. You might watch porn. By masturbating with your partner you are going to be able to enjoy each other's bodies while masturbating. Your partner might just prefer this if she is a woman. Just like woman don't quite know how men like to be touched, men don't know how women like it either. By masturbating in front of each other you can achieve intimacy without having to have intercourse.

You can also use mutual masturbation as a way to get erect before having sex. Try progressing to this level if you want to eventually be able to have penetrative sex with your partner. It is highly recommended that you at least try to penetrate your partner once you are erect. Another way you can use mutual masturbation to progress to sex is by masturbating your partner with your own fingers. Have her guide your movements, telling you where to go and what to do. By doing this, you are going to discover her body and where her pleasure lies. It is going to add a significant amount of intimacy to your relationship because you are going to be the one giving her pleasure.

Additionally, you can create a sexual connection by having your partner help you masturbate. You can guide her hands yourself, as this will teach her how to properly give you pleasure. It will at least be a step above simply looking at and touching each other while masturbating, and is an important stepping stone to getting over your erectile dysfunction. You and your partner can also make the experience more erotic by rubbing lube or oil on each other. Once you have gotten yourself hard, have your partner put oil or lubricant on your penis for you. This has the added benefit of getting you used to her touch as well, which will make it easier to have sex later on.

You don't have to try to do this the very first time you and your partner are intimate. However, in the long run mutual masturbation should really be considered as a buildup to penetrative sex. This is because penetrative sex is the most intimate form of sex there can be. If you are unable to have it you are not deficient in any way, but you might be missing out on sex that is truly transcendent.

## Use Sex Toys

Sometimes, your partner just needs some sexual satisfaction from you rather than from themselves. It is a perfectly ordinary request, and fair considering they are a sexual being too. Hence, it is important to give you partner sexual pleasure using whatever tools you can. A great way to do this would be to use sex toys. Sex toys are great because they can actually substitute for your penis in a lot of ways, and in certain ways can even provide superior pleasure.

There are several sex toys that you could use in order to get your partner off. The most popular is probably a vibrator. By using a vibrator, you will be able to provide intense pleasure to your woman. By applying it to your woman's clitoris, you are going to be able to give her intense orgasms. The use of vibrators is extremely effective, and is actually a normal sexual practice. It is a misconception that woman derive pleasure from penetration. While there is an erotic quality to this act and penetration does indeed provide a great deal of pleasure, most women find it extremely difficult to achieve an orgasm while they are being penetrated.

This is because a woman's pleasure center is actually outside her vagina: the clitoris. Hence, even if you and your partner were having penetrative sex, you might still be using a vibrator to get her off. That's just the way things work sometimes! However, this does not mean that your use of the vibrator on her has to be restricted to her clitoris. You can use the vibrator in a variety of other ways. One very popular use of the vibrator is on her G spot.

Her G spot is located inside her vagina. It is actually roughly in the same part of her body as your prostate is in your own body. Hence, if you are familiar with prostate massages, you are going to have no trouble whatsoever discovering this part of her body. If you use the vibrator on her G spot, you are going to be able to give her truly incredible orgasms. Indeed, her orgasms will be far more pleasurable than they would ever have been had you been using your penis instead of a vibrator. This is because a vibrator provides the stimulation of intense vibration aside from the thrusting motion that you are using it for.

If you want to get really kinky you can use two vibrators at the same time. One can be used on her clitoris, and the other one can be used on her G spot. By using two vibrators at once you are going to give her orgasms like she has never felt before! There is a cornucopia of other sex toys that you can use as well. One great example is an anal plug.

By putting an anal plug into your partners anus, you can provide intense stimulation to her. The act is intensely erotic and also tends to feel quite naughty as does anything that has to do with the anus.

A great sex toy that you can use is a string of anal beads. These are a series of beads that are either strung together or form a single plastic rod. You will insert these beads into your partner's anus and use a vibrator on her clitoris. Once she is climaxing, you can pull the beads out of her anus to push her orgasms to another level entirely! You can also use vibrators and anal beads on yourself. Remember, your prostate is extremely sensitive, and by stimulating it you can induce powerful orgasms within yourself.

You must use thinner vibrators than you would be using on your partner's vagina. Having your partner do it for you can make the experience a lot more erotic, and will probably end up giving even more powerful orgasms than you were expecting to have. You can also use anal beads on yourself while you are masturbating. Simply masturbate in front of your partner and have her keep a finger on the beads. Once you are about to achieve climax, have her pull the beads out in one movement. This is going to stimulate your prostate intensely. You are going to feel a sudden shock to the prostate with each bead that brushes up against it.

This can help you to enjoy far more stimulating orgasms. Additionally, your partner will be involved in the process of giving you pleasure. This is extremely important. Sometimes your partner would want to be the one who is giving you pleasure. It just feels good to know that the pleasure is coming from something one is doing to one's partner. By involving your partner in this way you will be able to enjoy sex together. Additionally, if you are in a same sex relationship, anal beads can become a great way for you and your partner to enjoy each other's bodies. You can use vibrators on each other as well in order to bring intimacy to the sex.

Hence, by using sex toys you will be able to have excellent sex without having to get erect at all.

## Sexting and Phone Sex

This is a great way to keep sex in your lives even if the two of you are extremely busy. It is important to keep the sex alive even if you are unable to meet each other. By using your cell phones, you can create a level of deep intimacy before having to actually get down to having sex. This is quite important, because having actual sex may be a very stressful experience for you. When you get into bed with a new partner, you might be under a lot of pressure to perform. You already know what pressure does to someone suffering from erectile dysfunction.

As a result of this pressure, it is going to be absolutely impossible for you to get erect during this first encounter. The best thing to do if this is the case is to "soften the blow" as it were.

By engaging in sexting and phone sex you are going to get used to your partner's sexual preferences and body without having to be under pressure to perform for her. Since you are simply getting images while sexting, getting hard won't be a problem for you if the erectile dysfunction you are suffering from is not severe and caused by biological anomalies. Sexting, hence, is the very first tier of gaining intimacy. Once you and your partner have sexted a little, you can move onto phone sex. Phone sex is a great way to take your intimacy to the next level. This is because you can actually hear each other's voices, and will be able to see the effect you are having on each other.

You can also respond to what your partner wants you to do. You might be asked to send a picture of yourself, or your partner might ask you to engage in a fantasy with her. This will allow you to gain a deeper understanding of her sexual preferences. You can use phone sex to discuss your own sexual preferences as well. One very important thing that phone sex might be able to help with is actually talking to your partner about your erectile dysfunction. Since you are going to be able to discuss it in a safe space of your choosing, and if your partner's responses are not what you expected you can always cut the call, discussing it over the phone is a great way to break the news without having to go through the stress of a face-to-face conversation about something so embarrassing.

Once the two of you have gained an adequate level of intimacy, you can move onto some more advanced levels of virtual sex. This would be video calling. Phone sex is great, but after a certain point you need to be able to see your partner respond to your sexual preferences and requests. You would want to be able to actually see your partner doing what you tell them to, and your partner would most likely want the same from you too. By having sex over a video call, you can attain a much higher level of intimacy. There is only so much you can ascertain from a person's voice. Sometimes, movement is necessary to determine whether what you are doing is in line with what that person wants.

Seeing your partner move while pleasuring themselves is important because it allows you to align your own movements to theirs. The visual component of sex will facilitate a deeper understanding of each other's sexual natures, and is a lot more enjoyable from a purely hedonistic aspect. You can even start incorporating some of the previously mentioned techniques. Sex over a video call is already pretty close to mutual masturbation. You can take this to the next level by incorporating sex toys into it. By having your partner use sex toys on herself, you can give her increased pleasure by proxy.

There are a lot of sex toys that you can use that will bridge the digital divide between you two. Certain sex toys and vibrators come with apps that allow them to be remotely accessed. Hence, you can be sitting in the comfort of your own home and giving your partner intense pleasure over a video call. This does not just remove the need for an erection, it makes the entire process of meeting each other unnecessary for a time. You can save the actual sex for later, while enjoying each other with through a screen for a period of time. Bear in mind that video calling is a big step up from phone sex. With video calling, a lot of the masks you might be able to wear while having phone sex will be gone. You will, literally, naked in front of your partner, or at least in a situation where your partner will be able to see you.

This involves a level of vulnerability that you might not be ready for. You might video call your partner and be unable to get erect, in spite of the fact that you were fully able to over phone sex. There is no shame in this, it is just a natural part of your erectile dysfunction. You are essentially under pressure to perform while on a video call. This is why you will suffer from performance anxiety, which will end up making it very difficult for you to get erect.

Use video sex only when you are ready. Once you start using it, sex practices such as mutual masturbation won't be far behind. You can use sexting, phone sex and video sex as stepping stones to mutual masturbation, which in itself is a stepping stone to getting over your erectile dysfunction and having penetrative sex. You can even use these practices in the gaps between your actual sex encounters. It will help you and your partner to maintain the intimacy you have fought so hard to achieve, despite the fact that you have not met each other in a long time.

## Oral Sex

If there is a single sex practice that you should engage in while you are suffering from erectile dysfunction, it is oral sex. This is because it's just a great way for you to give your partner pleasure. The problem with a lot of the aforementioned techniques and methods that you can use is that they involve some kind of barrier between you and your partner. Sexting, phone sex and video sex all involve sex through a digital wall of sorts. Additionally, having sex via mutual masturbation is pretty distant too. You just aren't getting the same level of intimacy you would be getting if you were to have penetrative sex.

Even using sex toys is sometimes not adequate. Although it can provide a great deal of pleasure for you and your partner, using sex toys is still artificial sex. Sometimes your partner would want a more organic touch to the sex you two are having. The best way to bring this touch of realness to your sex life is by engaging in oral sex. Oral sex is far superior to simply touching or masturbating your partner because it involves the use of your tongue. Your tongue is a lot more efficient and getting your woman to climax than your fingers are, probably because of the way it is built. There are several ways in which you can make oral sex a regular part of you and you're partner's sex life.

The key to oral sex is how you use your tongue. You need to press your tongue flat on your partner's clitoris. Make sure it is not flexed or hard. Your partner would enjoy it if your tongue is nice and soft. Once your soft tongue is place flat on your partner's clitoris, you can move it around in circles. This would provide enormous stimulation to the clitoris and would probably result in incredibly intense orgasms. You can get your fingers into it too. While you are giving your partner oral sex, you can penetrate her with your finger as well. Simultaneously stimulating her clitoris with your tongue along with her G spot with your fingers is a great way to give her amazing orgasms. This would be far superior to using vibrators because your partner would be getting her pleasure from an actual part of your body rather than a mechanical object.

A further level of oral sex would be to penetrate your partner's vagina with your tongue. This is rather difficult to do and can be quite uncomfortable for you but it is an intensely erotic experience for your partner for the sole reason that it will show her how committed you are to pleasuring her. The key is to start slow. You don't want to rush into things, and your partner certainly won't appreciate it. Savor her as you pleasure her, she will feel the tenderness with which you are pleasuring her and this will translate into her own pleasure.

It is also important to keep in mind that the clitoris is essentially a female version of a penis. This means that a lot of the things that you find pleasurable, she will also find pleasurable if you do it to her clitoris. Hence, apply some of the techniques that you find enjoyable and you might be surprised at how much she enjoys it. Just remember to try gentler versions of these techniques because a clitoris is vastly more sensitive than your penis. If you really want to get kinky, you can engage in anilingus. This involves stimulating your partner's anus with your tongue. You can just stimulate the edge of her anus and it would provide her with quite intense pleasure. Your partner can even do it to you if you are so inclined!

If you are having sex with a male partner, there are several techniques you can use in order to give him a pleasurable experience with oral sex. A good idea would be to stimulate the head of his penis with your tongue. The head of his penis is home to large cluster of nerves. Hence, is you pleasure this part of his penis, he is going to feel it more intensely than he would otherwise. Try to move your tongue around in a circle around the head of his penis.

If you really want to give him some intense pleasure, you can focus on the area just beneath the head of his penis. This would be the skin that connects the head of his penis to the rest of it. If you gently stimulate this area, he is going to end up having enormously pleasurable orgasms. He might just climax without even realizing he was close, such is the intensity of pleasure he can get from this area. You can also engage in other activities, such as gently stimulating his scrotums with your lips or tongue. This can be very pleasurable for your partner, and would greatly increase the level of intimacy that the two of you enjoy.

One thing you should keep in mind while giving your male partner oral sex is never to get teeth involved. Keep in mind what it's like to receive oral sex yourself. Anything you like is probably going to translate well to him. You can also give anilingus a try with your male partner. This is a very kinky activity and your partner will surely love it just as much as you do. Try rimming the edge of his anus with your tongue whilst simultaneously masturbating him. The twin sensations can result in excellent orgasms for your partner.

All in all, by applying oral sex techniques you can provide your partner with intimate pleasure in spite of your inability to get erect. In fact, a lot of the techniques described here are those that would be used by someone even if they were able to get erect because they are much more effective at providing women pleasure than penetration.

## BDSM

BDSM is a great way to bring some spice into your sex life. It is also rather enjoyable for you if you suffer from erectile dysfunction, because if you act dominant to your partner you probably won't even really need to penetrate her. The key here is to communicate. You and your partner should sit down and talk about what you want. If your partner wants you to be submissive, explain to her your sexual dysfunction. It probably won't matter either way, because your partner would want you to be submissive to her and would thus find your erectile dysfunction rather erotic.

There are a variety of ways in which you can spice up your sex life using BDSM techniques. One rather popular way is to use handcuffs. These wouldn't be the uncomfortable variety that police officers would use on convicted felons. Rather, they would fluffier handcuffs, covered in fur to make them comfortable. The fur will also provide a tickling sensation, which will increase your partner's sensitivity in bed. You can also tie your partner up with ropes. Ropes great to use if you want something that will hold, something that will prevent your partner from moving entirely. You will then be able to pleasure her using any of the aforementioned techniques and would thus be able to be in control of the situation.

The benefit here is that you are no longer under pressure to perform. You have your partner entire under your control, and this means that she cannot talk back to you. It is an intensely erotic way to have sex and will probably help a great deal with your erectile dysfunction. Apart from tying her up or otherwise restraining, you can use intense vibrators on her clitoris. While she is tied up, the effect of the vibrator will be much increased. The sensation of being unable to move will increase the intensity of pleasure, and the feeling of the rope will make her more susceptible to even the slightest touch.

One of the best ways to provide her pleasure while she is tied up is to tickle her. This is a form of sexual torture that results in a high level of intimacy. Tickling tends to illicit uncontrolled reactions from the person being tickled. This is why, when you tickle your partner, you are going to end up feeling intense love towards her, and this will help make the sex more intense and enjoyable.

In order to add more spice to your sex with BDSM, you can also blindfold your partner. This will help because it will completely take the pressure off you. She will be unable to see you, and the feeling of being tied up coupled with her temporary blindness will make everything you do to her far more erotic than it is. Even the touch of your breath on her ear will end up making her shudder while she is in this position. Since she is so easy to please while she is like this, you are going to be able to pleasure her without worrying about your performance. You might be surprised to learn about how little your erectile dysfunction matters. When the pressure is relieved, you are going to end up getting hard without realizing it.

You can also engage in submissive behavior in order to alleviate the problems caused by erectile dysfunction. The major benefit of this is that you are not going to be the active participant. Rather, you are going to be submissive to a dominant partner. As a result, she is going to be the one telling you what to do. When the pressure is off your shoulders to perform, when you are put in a situation where the only thing you have to do is follow instructions, you will find that it is a lot easier to get erect than it was before.

You can even encourage your partner to tie you up or handcuff you. Since you will be unable to move and are essentially a passive participant in sex, you will not have to worry about what to do to please your partner. Being in such a passive position makes the whole process of sex much easier for you, and a lot less stressful.

Just keep in mind that you have to communicate each other's desires to one another. Just because you are submissive in bed does not mean that you are in any way less of a man, or that you are somehow supposed to be submissive in every aspect of your life. Sex is supposed to be restricted to the bedroom. Outside of it you can be just as dominant as you have to be. Inside it, however, you can do whatever you need to in order to have sex. While engaging in BDSM, your partner is responsible for your safety if you are a sub. However, this does not mean that you need to keep your mouth shut if your partner is engaging in a sexual practice that you are not comfortable with. If what you are doing or what is being done to you is outside your comfort zone, be sure to tell your partner. Chances are, your partner just does not know that they are crossing a line.

Additionally, being a dominant sexual partner in bed does not mean that you have to cause your partner pain. Whips are a definite part of BDSM, but this does not mean that pain is essential to getting over your erectile dysfunction. Being dominant in bed is not an excuse to hurt your partner either. Sex is always consensual, as is everything that has anything to do with sex. Just remember to keep it safe and to only go to places where both your partners have discussed before. This is primarily a way to get over your erectile dysfunction and allow you and your partner to enjoy sex in spite of the fact that you are unable to get erect.

## *Masturbating with Your Prostate*

If you are experiencing the kind of erectile dysfunction that comes from a faulty prostate or from some other biological problem, the aforementioned techniques might not work. Masturbation in particular would be difficult for you because you simply would not be able to get erect. For such situations, prostate massage is an excellent option. It can result in intense orgasms and can allow you and your partner to engage in actual sex with each other. There is a step by step process by which you can engage in a prostate massage either on your own or with your partner.

## Empty your Bowels

This is a very important part of the process. You would probably at any given time have feces in your rectum. Hence, when you insert your fingers into your anus to massage your prostate, you might end up touching your feces which is certainly not something that you would want to do. If your partner touches your feces it would completely kill the mood, which is understandable. Hence, in order to make the massage fun, it is essential that you empty your bowels before you do anything else.

## Take a Shower

Cleanliness is an essential part of prostate massages. Just to be sure that you are absolutely clean, take a shower taking special care to wash that particular part of your body. If you simply don't want to take a shower, you can just wash yourself down there instead. Just take special care to clean yourself out completely. A good idea would be to remove the hair from that area too. No matter how much you clean yourself, hair on your backside is going to be a major turn off for your partner. Remove the potential for disruption in your sex by removing the hair from that area.

## Cut Your Nails

If you are planning on giving yourself a prostate massage, it would be a good idea to trim your nails. This is because you might end up cutting or nicking yourself if you penetrate your anus with a finger that has long nails. If your partner is giving you a prostate massage, have her trim her nails. If she does not want to she can try wearing gloves while performing the massage. However, it is highly recommended that she cuts her nails, as a proper massage is done without gloves and is a great deal more pleasurable.

## Position Yourself

The best position to get to your prostate is with you on your back. Try tucking your knees into your chest, and placing a cushion under your lower back in order to facilitate easier entry. If this position isn't working for you, try out other positions. You can lie down on your side with a single knee raised (not the one that is one the bed). You can also try getting on all fours and curving your lower back. Every man is different, and finding out which position suits you is an important part of getting a good prostate massage.

## Lube Up

One thing that you need to keep in mind is that your anus is not really designed for taking in fingers or other objects, it is designed for expelling things. Hence, in order to ensure that you have an easy time finding your prostate, you need to use lubricant. Just add a few drops to your fingers or your partner's fingers if she is the one doing the prostate massage for you. You can even add lube to your anus if that is more comfortable for you. Once the lube has been applied, you are ready to insert your finger in.

## Put Your Finger In

This part is rather tricky because people tend to be a little overexcited while doing this. As a result, they end up thrusting their finger in too roughly and end up causing discomfort. Remember, this is masturbation. You are supposed to enjoy this.

When you put your finger in, do it as gently as possible. Feel your way inside slowly, do not force anything. Your anus will slowly open up to you if you are moving properly. If you take it slow, you will slowly feel any obstructions in your way move aside. The key here is to relax. If you are embarrassed or tense in any way, the muscles in your anus are going to clench. When they clench, it is going to become far more difficult for you to reach your prostate.

The lube should help here. Your anus does not have natural lubricants the way a vagina does, but the lube will compensate for that. If your partner is the one who is penetrating your anus, make sure to communicate with them. Ensure that they know whether you are comfortable or not. Remember that they are not feeling what you are feeling, so the clearer you are about your level of comfort the easier it will be for both of you to enjoy the experience.

You or your partner should slide the finger in until the second knuckle. This is usually how much penetration is required in order to reach the prostate; however, the exact location differs from person to person. Try out different areas and angles, tell your partner to feel around inside you for the right spot.

Once he or she hits the spot, you are going to feel a rather different sensation. Apart from the feeling of them being inside you, you are going to start feeling a light buzzing sensation and are going to be filled with an overpowering urge to contract the muscles of your anus. This is natural, and is similar to the response that women have when you touch their G spot.

However, if you clench your muscles your anus might end up pushing your partner's finger out with the exact same peristalsis it uses to push feces out. If your partner tries to fight against the peristalsis, they might end up injuring you slightly. Hence, it is better that you try your best to avoid clenching the muscles when they hit the prostate.

This will take some practice to do because the sensation when they touch the prostate is going to be intense. The first few times you are inevitably going to push your partner's finger out. Eventually, though, when you get used to the sensation you are going to be better able to avoid the clenching of your muscles. This is why it is recommended that you try to practice on yourself before engaging in this activity with a partner. Once you have discovered your own sexual preferences during this activity, it will become easier for you to guide your partner. Knowledge of one's own body is always supposed to come first.

The finger going in should be doing so with the palm facing up. This is because in order to actually reach the prostate, the finger will have to curl upwards. Once you or your partner's finger is inside, have them curl it upwards and you will feel it brushing against your prostate. If you have practiced keeping your muscles loose, your partner will be able to stimulate your prostate quite frequently.

The sensation will increase to the point where you will begin to feel the pleasure spread across your backside. This blooming of pleasure will spread upwards to your lower back and down the back of your thighs. Unlike with regular masturbation, your groin or penis is the last place the pleasure will reach. It is hard to really know when you have achieved orgasm via your prostate. The climax does not arrive suddenly as with real masturbation, but this process does leave you satisfied. It is thus a rather useful substitute for masturbation and can be a great way for you and your partner to have sex in spite of your erectile dysfunction.

## Use Sex Toys

You already know how you can use vibrators and butt plugs in order to stimulate your prostate. Prostate stimulation is also a great way to have sex in a same sex relationship. If your partner penetrates your anus, he can stimulate your prostate gland with his penis. This is standard sex practice among homosexual males, but a lot of people don't know that even the receiving partner, or "bottom", can receive sexual pleasure during sex. Hence, erectile dysfunction can prove to be an easily solvable problem if you are gay.

This same basic principle can translate over to heterosexual relationships too. There is a sex toy called a "strap on" which is essentially a belt of sorts on which a dildo is attached. This can allow your female partner to penetrate you and stimulate your prostate gland. This is a perfectly legitimate way to have sex and can allow you and your partner to have sex in an intimate manner. It can also really turn the tables in your sex life, as you would be the receiving partner for a change! You can also use strap ons yourself. If you suffer from erectile dysfunction, your main problem is that you cannot have penetrative sex with your partner. As a result, you might feel that you are not able to achieve the same level of intimacy that other people might have.

By using a strap on you can solve this problem. In both heterosexual and homosexual relationships, if you are suffering from erectile dysfunction, you can easily have penetrative sex using a strap on. It removes the need to get an erection entirely, and can allow you to be deeply intimate with your partner. It is important to remember here that the accumulated stress of being unable to satisfy your partner for a long period of time can be an enormous contributing factor in erectile dysfunction. This is an area where using a strap on can help you immensely. By using a strap on, you can alleviate some of the sexual frustration that might have built up within your partner due to the fact that you are unable to get an erection.

Since your partner will be satisfied with you, sexually speaking, you will be under less pressure during sex. You might be able to get an erection without even realizing it!

In this way, using a strap on can be an important stepping stone to penetrative sex with your penis. It can even be considered the final stepping stone. After sexting, phone sex, video sex, mutual masturbation and the use of toys, you can start having sex that is very close to actual penetrative sex using this technique. You will then just be a baby step away from overcoming your erectile dysfunction. You can even change things up in bed. You can use a butt plug on yourself while penetrating your partner with a strap on. You can use a vibrating butt plug that will stimulate your prostate so that you get pleasure during sex as well. You can put anal beads in and have your partner pull them out when she is climaxing so that you can feel pleasure with her.

The possibilities are endless with sex. Just because you have erectile dysfunction doesn't mean that your life has ended. A normal relationship may be impossible, but in today's modern day and age normal no longer exists. With so many options, you may not have a sex life that you can classify as "normal", but you will certainly have one that is fulfilling and enjoyable for both and your partner.

Bear in mind that if the reason for your erectile dysfunction is low blood supply or excess fat, using a strap on will not help you get erect. This would only work if the stress of an unsatisfied partner is keeping you from getting erect. However, using a strap on will allow you to penetrate your partner with an artificial penis, and thrust in the exact same motion that you would if you were using your penis. Hence, in such situations strap on may be slightly less useful, but they would still be incredibly useful nonetheless.

# Chapter Seven: Could a Sex Therapist Help?

Sex therapists seem to be everywhere these days – on chat shows, online, on the radio, and even in your high street. You may be living next door to a sex therapist and not even know it! So, what is a sex therapist, what do they do, and can they help with erectile dysfunction? Here are some of the answers to your questions. Only you can decide if a sex therapist is appropriate in your particular case, and this chapter should help you to make that decision.

## What is a sex therapist?

A properly qualified sex therapist – and that's the only type you should consider using - is likely to have a background in relationship counseling, psychiatry, psychology or clinical social work. They may even have a medical background, but they will have received specialist training in order to be recognized as a sex therapist qualified to advise individuals or couples on problems within their relationships that are sexually related in some way.

Put simply, a sex therapist treats sex problems with science and an open mind, in the specialized manner that is often required in such cases. Personal opinion and experience are not usually likely to influence the way they work with their patients, and each new case is approached with an open mind, but also with several scientifically proven solutions in mind. Although the treatment is tailored to the individual, it is based on years of experience in the field, and scientific back up. Most sex therapists have a much more detailed knowledge of human physiology as it is affected by sexuality, and all the processes the body goes through before, during and after sexual intercourse. In fact, a really good sex therapist may have more expert knowledge of this particular area of physiology than many medical practitioners.

A sex therapist is not a snake oil salesman or a prostitute or escort under a more job polite description. It's not like in some porn films, where the sex therapist jumps into bed with one, two or several of his or her clients, and everyone's sexual problems are resolved as if by magic with the cameras rolling. In fact, most sex therapy revolves around talk and advice. In a few – very rare – cases, a surrogate partner therapist may be used. We'll take a look at that option later in this chapter, because it's something totally different.

## What to expect from a sex therapist?

In the initial session, your sex therapist will want you to do most of the talking, so he or she can determine whether the cause of your problem is physical, psychological or a combination of both. Questions will be asked, and you'll need to answer them as fully and as honestly as you can. Depending on the exact details of your personal case, it may take more than one session to complete this important first step.

This detailed assessment will help the sex therapist to formulate a plan of action for you, and decide how often you need to attend therapy sessions. The therapist may suggest that your partner attends some or all of the sessions with you, or you may attend on your own. You will not be expected to do anything against your wishes, and the atmosphere should be relaxed and friendly, to allow you to open up to your therapist and work together to solve your problems.

Part of the therapy will involve doing exercises at home between the sessions, either alone or with your partner. These will be formulated to help you understand your body and your sexuality, and enhance your self-confidence and sexual awareness. You should remember – and your therapist should remind you regularly – that sex is supposed to be an enjoyable, pleasurable experience, and the sessions will be geared towards that achievement. Some of the exercises may not seem to have much point, but remember this is a scientific treatment program, and there is a reason for everything you are asked to do. If you don't understand something, ask your therapist to explain, because you need to work together on this if you are to get maximum benefit from the sessions.

You will need to provide a detailed history of your sex life to date. This is not salacious interest on the part of the therapist – it's an excellent way to pinpoint when problems started, and in some cases, why. You'll also need to talk about masturbation, because in a lot of cases of erectile dysfunction – particularly those involving younger men – there is no problem achieving or maintaining an erection, it just happens when they are with a partner. This may mean that performance anxiety is exacerbating your problem, and your therapy will be geared to address this, and any other issues that transpire during the initial assessment.

Everything you say to your therapist is and will always remain confidential, so be open and honest, and answer all questions as fully as you can. Talking in this way helps you to understand why you are having problems maintaining erections, as well as teasing out long-buried stuff that you thought you'd forgotten but which may still be impacting on your life, even after many years. It's all very cathartic, and it can help your therapist to formulate the most appropriate and effective program for your needs. Don't be ashamed and hold back on anything – it may be a cliché, but your therapist really has heard it all before. He or she will not be shocked by your revelations, so open up, and let it all out in the presence of someone who is highly trained to help you work through your problems and move on with your life and your sex life.

Although the atmosphere is meant to be relaxed and intimate, inviting confidences, the therapist will not touch you, because what goes on in the office is based around talk, not bodily contact. It's against the professional code of practice to touch clients, and this will be explained to you at the outset. It makes sense when you think about it – it would be only too easy for the client to develop an unhelpful and inappropriate attachment to his therapist, given the nature of the secrets he's shared.

The therapist is also likely to ask about your general life outside the bedroom, because he or she needs to build a picture of you as a complete person in order to offer the best counseling and advice for your particular case. Although sex therapy is a science like medicine, the difference is that it's not also tailored to the individual. There may only be one way to remove an appendix, for example, but there are countless ways to approach the treatment of erectile dysfunction within the scientific framework.

And it may be that some of the exercises you are asked to do have nothing to do with sex at all. Nevertheless, they are geared towards helping you to attain a more satisfying sex life. For example, if it emerges that you have a poor body image, you may be advised to join a gym or fit some extra exercise into your routine. Or it might be suggested that you try to build more intimacy with your partner in various ways – maybe by having an evening where you sit and hold hands, talk to each other about your dreams for the future or even touch or caress each other, without attempting to have sex.

One very successful way to re-establish lost intimacy is to lie in bed together naked, touching and cuddling, but not attempting foreplay or sex. Often, the simple act of removing the pressure to have sex can be a big help in solving issues of erectile dysfunction, so the therapist may even advise you not to have sex for a certain period of time, and if this is the case, you should respect the advice, because he or she has been dealing with this sort of stuff for a long time. When the therapist thinks you are ready to have successful and fulfilling sexual intercourse, you will be the first to know!

Other 'homework' may include non-sexual touching exercises and recommended reading. The whole process is geared to help you to get to know yourself and your sexuality on a deeper level, so that you can understand what has happened to you and why, and then work through it and take your relationship to the next, happier and more intimate level.

Many sex therapists say that the saddest thing about their profession is that couples and individuals treat sex therapy as the 'last chance saloon,' when so many of the problems they are presented with can be resolved very quickly and simply, even though they initially appear insurmountable to their clients. Most sexual problems do have a solution, but too often, anger and resentment has built up and it may be too late to save the relationship.

Relationship counseling is a natural part of sex therapy – your therapist needs to determine whether something in the relationship is causing or contributing to your erectile dysfunction. In fact, you can expect to cover all aspects of your life and feelings with your sex therapist. Very often, talking about things that have been bottled up for too long – especially things related to sex and intimacy – is a liberating experience for the client, and a revealing one, and you may often discover ways to improve your situation, simply by talking about them with someone who is giving you their undivided attention. If other methods have failed, maybe sex therapy is worth some of your time and effort in your quest to conquer erectile dysfunction.

## *Surrogate Partner Therapy (SPT)*

Surrogate Partner Therapy was the brainchild of American sex experts Masters & Johnson, and it's been around for around 60 years, although it's only recently become more mainstream, due to media attention and movies like *The Sessions*, which dealt with what has up to know been seen as something that's little short of legalized prostitution, or an affair with a veneer of respectability. However, used in the right way and for the right people, it can help men to overcome erectile dysfunction.

A sex therapist does not offer sex as part of the client's therapy. Indeed, professional ethics and common sense decree that no body contact should take between client and therapists during consultations. However, another aspect of sex therapy, which is usually used in conjunction with conventional therapy sessions involve using a surrogate partner who will perform sexual and intimate acts with you as part of the therapy. Not every client is a suitable candidate for this, and not every case is appropriate for surrogate partner therapy.

This is no regular affair, and it's nothing like an encounter with a prostitute – it's a businesslike arrangement in which a highly trained surrogate will work with a client to address and treat their sexual problems in conjunction with conventional sex therapy. At the same time, the surrogate and client form a real relationship and develop the level of intimacy and sharing that is necessary for the surrogate to help the client to achieve his sexual aims and enjoy happy, healthy and fulfilling relationships in the future.

The surrogate may or may not interact sexually with the client, but when that happens, it's not about pleasure in the moment – it's about dealing with the sexual problem, and helping the client through it by educating him about his body, his sexual and emotional responses and using both structured and unstructured exercises and techniques to overcome the issue of erectile dysfunction.

However, SPT is not all about sex – it's concerned with the whole spectrum of relationships – how you feel about your body, and how you can have a much better, happier and long-term relationship with your life partner or partners, with sex, but most of all, and most importantly, with yourself. It may be good to talk, but sometimes talk isn't enough, and people need practical experience in overcoming sex-related issues – if you want to put it a particular way, they need to be shown, rather than advised, how to overcome their sexual difficulties.

Working with a trained partner who is deeply aware of their own sexuality as well as having a specialized knowledge about giving and receiving pleasure can be very rewarding for some people. In the case of erectile dysfunction, this approach may work where others have failed, because there is no pressure to please, even if the pressure is self-imposed. This is a learning experience, and the client will be shown techniques and talked through why some things work and others do not.

SPT is a combination of scientifically developed sexual exercises aimed at rethinking the attitude and developing couples' communication so that everything in the bedroom is geared towards mutual pleasure and enjoyment, rather than seeing orgasm as the end objective, and New Age and Eastern thinking on self-awareness and relaxation techniques. You learn to connect mind and body through meditation, relaxation and breathing exercises, combined with practical techniques designed to enhance enjoyment for both partners. This brings about a new self-confidence that is not confined to the bedroom but radiates into all areas of the client's life.

The successful surrogate partner will work to build the same level of intimacy and commitment that exists in regular relationships. This may involve various exercises in touching sexually, sensually and even non-sexually, as well as encouragement and training in social skills, and learning to please a partner and accept intimacy and pleasure unselfconsciously.

Some SPTs claim 85% success in cases of erectile dysfunction, and claim to succeed where conventional therapy and medical intervention have previously failed. Ensure that your potential surrogate has been trained to International Professional Surrogate Association standards and ask lots of questions before committing to an expensive program of treatment. You will also work with a regular sex therapist, and between the three of you, you will decide on boundaries, goals, and the length of your relationship with your surrogate. Yes, it's expensive, but you may consider it money well spent if it solves your problems. However, not every man is a suitable candidate for Surrogate Partner Therapy, so it may be better to talk to a conventional sex therapist before pursuing that treatment option.

While sex therapy is not for everyone, it is a viable option for treating erectile dysfunction, because it concentrates on the sexual aspect of your life while also encompassing your relationships and lifestyle. It can be initially embarrassing to discuss such intimate matters, but you could find the experience both empowering and effective. Cost may be a determining factor, since sex therapy, and particularly surrogate partner therapy, can be expensive, and is not usually covered national health services or regular health insurance policies. However, if other options have failed, you may want to try some form of sex therapy to address your erectile dysfunction issues.

# Chapter Eight: Is Lack of Confidence Causing ED?

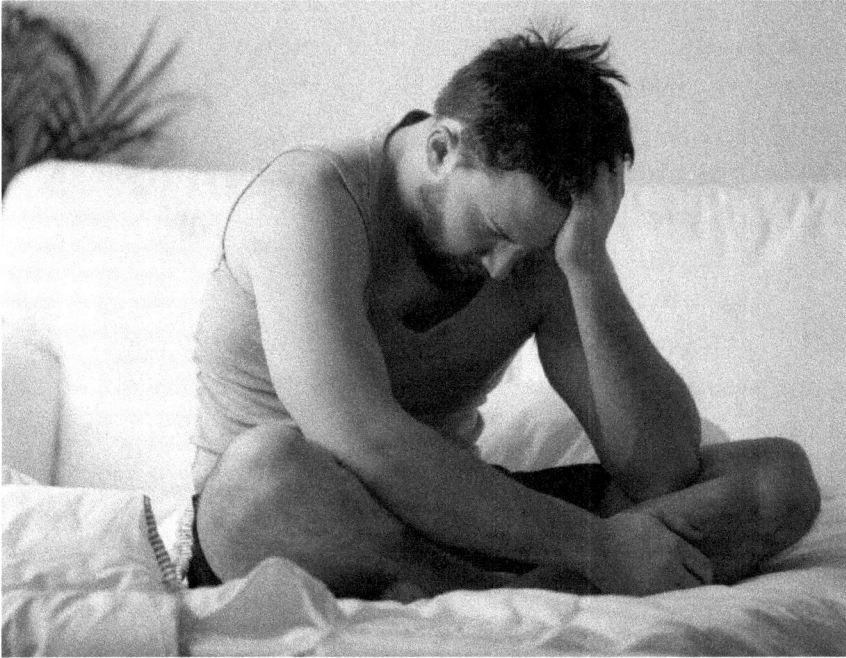

So far, this book has examined various physical causes of erectile dysfunction, and discussed some of the treatment options, including diet and lifestyle changes. But sometimes, there may not be a physical cause for the problem. If you're in your 30s, fit and well, with great vascular function and you're not carrying any extra weight or suffering from a chronic condition, yet you still have problems achieving and maintaining an erection, maybe you need to look beyond the physical.

Sometimes, lack of confidence can be the problem. It doesn't necessarily have to be sexually related either. It may stem from a fear of not being good enough for someone you care deeply about. You want to please them so much – not just sexually, but in every way possible. You want to be a friend, lover and provider. They are the most important person in your life, and you want to be the most important person in theirs. The problem is, you want it so badly, that you doubt your ability to deliver.

You may have a great job that pays well, that you enjoy, and you're good at, as well as being highly regarded by your boss and colleagues. You may even have a lovely home, and no money worries. You're a good-looking guy, not carrying too much weight, and you've still got all your own teeth. And you have the right work/life balance, so what's stopping you from enjoying a great relationship with the woman you love? Frankly, you are! You're trying to be the perfect partner in every way, and there is no such animal. Nobody is perfect. All anyone can do, whatever their advantages or disadvantages, is to do their best. The problem is, you may feel that your best just isn't good enough, and that's when the problems start.

It may not even start with sexual performance – chances are that everything in the bedroom is rosy at first. It's as you get to know each other better and move towards commitment that confidence issues may arise. The thing is, when a relationship gets to this stage, you start to think about the future. Until now, you've been enjoying each other's company – and hopefully each other's bodies – and all the thinking you've done is about how much you enjoy being together and how you can't wait for the next time. Once you start thinking about making a life together, anxieties and doubts start to creep in. Not about your partner – you're as sure as you can be that she's the one. Your doubts revolve around yourself, and your ability to be the partner she wants and deserves.

The way to get over this is to focus your thoughts on something else, other than yourself and your perceived failings. It can be a person or a thing, as long as it stops you thinking about yourself and therefore undermining your confidence even further. Some psychologists recommend losing yourself in a logic puzzle, or a difficult cryptic crossword or Sudoku. If you're not into puzzles, try burying yourself in a really good book, or even a video game. The important thing is that every time you feel your thoughts turning inwardly, you distract them before you get into that vicious cycle of doubt and anxiety, where you convince yourself that you're a failure, and it eventually becomes a self-fulfilling prophecy.

If you can get involved in something that holds your attention, you can break the cycle of negative thoughts and feelings. It may not feel like it, but you can actually control your thoughts and feelings, and take them in another direction. While it's all too easy to slide into a spiral of negative thinking that can result in erectile dysfunction, it's more difficult to train yourself to think positively, and turn your attitude around. Difficult – but by no means impossible.

The problem is, even if negativity doesn't start in the bedroom, that's where it's likely to end up, unless you can break the cycle. Men – unlike women – are not good about talking about their problems, especially when it comes to sex, because so much is invested in sexual performance, as far as most men are concerned. If there are problems in the bedroom, they see themselves as failures – no matter how successful they are in other areas of their lives, men who can't satisfy themselves and their partners sexually consider themselves to be failures. When it comes down to it, the good job, the nice house, the fancy car and the money in the bank count for nothing if they can't get an erection.

There are only two requirements for an erection – you need to be aroused, and you also need to be relaxed. If you are lacking in confidence, for whatever reason, you are not likely to be relaxed, and if your self-confidence issues have been ongoing for some time, you probably can't get aroused either.

## *Things You Can Do To Increase Self-Confidence*

Many people don't realize it but self-confidence is like physical muscles – it can be developed through training. It can get better with continuous use or get weak as it's left unused. The following are good ways to exercise your self-confidence muscles and develop them even more:

• Continue learning new things. One of the ways you can feel confident is by knowing things that most other people don't, including sexual tips and tricks. Who says learning can't be fun, eh?

• Step out of yourself and be a better person by doing something good for other people. How does this help develop self-confidence? By regularly thinking and doing something good for other people, you train yourself to be selfless and the less self-centered you become, the less conscious you become about your perceived "shortcomings", which lessens your tendency to be down on yourself.

• Hit the weights at the gym. If you want to look as buffed and macho as Hugh Jackman, Ryan Gosling and Ryan Reynolds, skip the marathons and hit the weights. You don't build muscles with cardio – you do it with resistance training. I know it sounds superficial but hey, looking buffed and macho can do a lot to boost self-confidence.

• Get out there and meet people even if you're an introvert. One of the best ways to overcome fear is by facing them head on and for most men who lack self-confidence, one of their greatest fears is reaching out and meeting new people. Confident people aren't afraid to make new friends and making new friends does wonders to boost self-confidence. So next time you're at a social event, get out of your comfort zone and meet new people.

- Know what matters most to you. There are times that not knowing what you value most can lead to low self-esteem. How? By being all over the place, you may spread yourself too thin to achieve anything significant. By knowing what matters most to you, you can focus your time, effort and resources on those priorities and increase your chances of achieving meaningful things, which can do wonders for self-confidence.

- Identify things that are harmful to you and your self-esteem that aren't really needed in your life and make an effort to get rid of them. Are you in an emotionally draining relationship with a girlfriend? Break up with her and find your joy elsewhere. Life's too short to be too preoccupied with unnecessary emotional stress and self-esteem bubble bursters.

- Do something you absolutely fear. Just keep it to safe and healthy ones, ok? Overcoming serious fears help bump up self-confidences several notches. For example, people who have had near-death experiences tend to become more sociable and confident knowing that they cheated something that most other people fear most – death. Try eating an exotic dish that most people absolutely fear eating, go bungee jumping or approach that hot chick sitting at the bar to introduce yourself and get her digits.

- Do some self-searching to identify thought patterns or habits that normally cause you to feel unconfident about yourself. After you've done so, imagine that someone close to you is thinking the same way and as a result, experience low self-esteem. How would you talk them out of feeling that way? Do the same to yourself.

- Identify the things that really make you intellectually and emotionally come alive and make time to regularly indulge in them. Often times, doing the things that make you alive translate directly to higher self-esteem.

- Step out of the roles you play in life that you're squeezing into just to please other people but aren't really cut out for. If for example, you're trying to be an insurance salesman because your parents expect you to become one just like your dad but being one isn't really your thing, there's nothing wrong in dropping it in favor of something you really want to do and know are more equipped to succeed in. Continuously trying to conform to others' expectations of you at the expense of what you really want (assuming what you want isn't sinful or illegal) is a sure-fire way to emasculate yourself and is the figurative equivalent of being neutered.

- Develop the skill of catching yourself every time you say or think that you're not good enough, talented enough or endowed enough to succeed. Learn to replace those self-depreciating scripts with confidence building ones. One way to help you do this is by regularly basking in the memories of past successes. As long as you don't overdo it, you remind yourself that you are worth something and that you are capable of achieving things, which can significantly help you have a healthy self-confidence.

- Stop the habit of making important decisions without deliberately thinking through them. By thinking through such decisions and being deliberate with them, you reduce your risk of making wrong ones and consequently, increase your chances of making good and successful ones. Thinking through includes acknowledging your concerns and doubts in order to have as much of your decision bases covered. There's a difference between being pessimistic and being pragmatic. Be the latter, not the former.

- Stop beating yourself up over past mistakes such as wrong decisions, inability to perform as expected or passing up on a great opportunity because doing so won't make things better but will only make them worse. The best thing to do is learn from them and realize that everybody makes mistakes every now and then. When similar situations crop up, you'll be more confident knowing what caused you to screw up a similar situation in the past and that you're now in a position to avoid making the same mistake.

- Don't confuse being scared with not being confident. Even the most confident people can still be scared at times. I know of a person who preaches to crowds of thousands every week and still feel so nervous before going up on stage that sometimes he pukes before going to the auditorium. It's ok to be scared – it's an acknowledgment that you're not perfect. What's not ok is not to be confident.

- There will always be people who'll make you feel unsure of yourself with the things they say to and about you. There's a difference between constructive feedback and outright putting you down and you don't have to put up with the latter. Either tell them to stop putting you down or leave them. You'll be much better without them anyway.

- This may sound unrelated but trust me it is – flirt! Why? The better you get at it with women, the more confident you'll feel about yourself. Trust me.

- Be vulnerable to others. Being vulnerable allows you to overcome one of the biggest fears for most people – rejection. As you master the art of vulnerability, you don't just master the fear of rejection, you'll find that people will draw closer to you and be vulnerable too. You have the side benefit of enjoying more intimate relationships on top of increased self-confidence.

- Be humble and admit it when you're wrong. Confidence for the sake of confidence is a fake one and won't last long. It's like building a mansion on sand. What you'd want is a self-confidence that sticks and lasts. Admitting your mistake has the same effect as being vulnerable – you let go of your fear of rejection and as a bonus, you earn other people's respect and confidence too.

- Regularly see yourself in your mind's eye (visualize) as the successful and confident person you want to be. Truth is, our subconscious minds are the ones responsible for our regular behavior and feelings and it can't distinguish what's real or not. By visualizing your successful self often, you feed the idea of a successful you to your subconscious mind and over time, it will act out that confident self you've fed it.

- Learn to ask for help. Why? You wont' be able to do everything by yourself. By enlisting the help of others, you'll be able to achieve more meaningful goals, which directly increase your self-confidence. Knowing you have other people to back you up in important tasks can also make you feel more confident about taking bigger responsibilities.

- Take risks. No meaningful achievements were ever accomplished without taking risks and the higher the risk, the bigger the potential success. If you want to be a successful person and feel more confident, you'll definitely have to be comfortable taking risks. Just take well-calculated ones though. Taking risks doesn't necessarily mean gambling your life and safety away.

- Spend more time with people who make you feel appreciated, important and significant. You can only go so far convincing yourself of such and the validation of others is a very powerful tool for building and increasing self-confidence.

- Fake it till you make it. Actions can go a long way towards influencing your thoughts and emotions. If you want to feel and think confident, start acting the part.

- Stop comparing yourself to others. It's a well-known fact that there will always be someone who'll be better at you at what you do best. As such, know that it's very counterproductive to compare yourself to other people, regardless if the people you're comparing yourself to are "superior" or "inferior" to you. The only person you should compare yourself to is yourself.

- Speak your mind during group discussions more often. For many people, speaking in front of many others can be quite a scary experience. If you deliberately go against your fear of speaking in public by speaking out your mind every time you're in a group, especially a large one such as a seminar or class, you weaken the fear and will start to experience a sense of self-confidence you've never experienced before. Face the fear to kill it and be more confident!

- Learn to value yourself for who you are and not who people want you to be. Live your life according to your values and beliefs and start experiencing unparalleled freedom from people's expectations, which will make you a truly confident person.

## *What Confident People Don't Do*

For many people, confidence is equal to being proud or self-centered. Nothing can be farther from the truth. The fact is, people who are truly confident about themselves don't go around bragging about themselves or tooting their own horns. If any, confident people are either thought of initially as shy or indifferent. Shy because they're often silent about their accomplishments knowing they don't have anything to prove. Indifferent because confident people couldn't care less about what goes on around them or about what others think of them.

To help you become more confident, here's a list of some of the things truly confident people don't do:

- They avoid humiliating or judging others because not only is it wrong, they are secure enough with who they are that they don't feel the need to put others down just bring themselves up. In fact, they do the opposite: they lift other people up because they're not insecure.
- They don't try to bring attention to themselves because again, they're secure with who they are that they don't feel the need to be noticed.
- They also don't try to dismiss any attention that's given to them freely. Because of the same sense of security, they're able to graciously and comfortably receive attention from others.
- They don't brag about themselves or whatever they've achieved. Why? Why not? They don't need others' approval to feel good about themselves so they don't feel the need to brag.
- They don't dismiss others' compliments about them and their achievements either. In fact, being confident in who they are allows them to comfortably receive and acknowledge other peoples' praises without letting those get into their heads.
- They're not critical. Because they're secure, they don't feel the need to criticize others and as such,

they ooze positivity and charisma, which attracts more people to them and make them feel even more confident.

- They don't just talk about themselves. An offshoot of being confident about one's identity and person is the ability to talk more about others than one's self. They are genuinely interested in others and it shows in them asking much about others and genuinely wanting to know others better and praise them. As such, confident people make for great conversationalists.

- They don't fuss over the small things. Because confident people are secure with themselves, they're also confident about being able to handle situations and thus don't make a fuss when things go wrong. Such confidence leads to a calmness in the face of challenges, whether big or small, which inspires the people around them to be as calm and collected.

- Confident people don't focus on things that aren't important. A big chunk of being confident is knowing what are the truly important things to focus on and as such, they're able to stick to what's really important and maximize their time, effort and resources.

- They don't break promises and commitments. Confident people know when to commit and promise and when not to because they know the things that they're truly capable of accomplishing. As such, confident people rarely overpromise and under deliver but usually under promise and over deliver. By doing the latter, they minimize the risk of broken promises and commitments.

# Conclusion

Erectile dysfunction or impotence is not a disease. It is a medical condition which can be caused by the various factors mentioned in this book. Therefore, one need not feel embarrassed, ashamed, guilty, or blame themselves for something that can be treated or cured. Millions of men suffer from this condition, yet the number of people actively seeking help is comparatively low. Though awareness has increased considerably in recent years, education about the condition is needed to help more men come out of their cocoon and seek the necessary help.

Awareness of the condition will help you realize that it is not something to be ashamed of and that it is not the end of a happy sex life. Hopefully you are aware of the various treatment options available now that you have read this book. Men can now take comfort in knowing that erectile dysfunction is not the end of manhood as they know it. You should not hesitate to consult a physician to have it taken care of in the initial stage. Get individualized treatment and feel free to consult about combination therapy depending upon your need.

Adopting a healthier lifestyle not only helps with this condition but also for a healthy life overall. As stated in the beginning, we are a species with intelligence and physical strength, yet one needs a happy sex life to balance every aspect of life. So, start making the changes you need to free yourself from this distressing condition. Do not hesitate to get your life back.

# Frequently Asked Questions

**Which Specialist doctor should I consult with when I present with the problem of erectile dysfunction?**

Kindly consult with a urologist if you sense the symptoms of or are already suffering from erectile dysfunction.

**Can alternative medicine cure erectile dysfunction?**

Yes, with your doctor's advice and recommendation, you may take alternative medicines such as: Nutritional supplements -, bioflavonoids, zinc, vitamin C, vitamin E, Amino acid arginine and flaxseed meal can improve erectile function. Herbal medicines- Moringa oleifera, Asian ginseng

**Does exercise help with erectile dysfunction?**

Yes, aerobic exercises are known to improve erectile dysfunction.

**Is Erectile Dysfunction a normal phenomenon of aging?**

No. you don't necessarily have ED as you grow older. Some men at old age still have normal erections. Although, as you age, you may observe that it would take your partner's long stimulation by romance and stroking you to initiate an erection.

## Is Viagra good for treating ED in Diabetics?

Yes, Viagra may be a successful therapy for erectile dysfunction in men, with a minimum of side effects.

## Is erectile dysfunction an STD?

No. Erectile dysfunction is not a sexually transmitted disease.

## Is premature ejaculation an erectile dysfunction?

No. Premature ejaculation is different from erectile dysfunction. In premature ejaculation, the sufferer does not have problem getting an erection suitable for sex whereas in erectile dysfunction, there is difficulty in having and maintaining an erection.

## What causes a erectile dysfunction?

There are many causes of Erectile Dysfunction. These include anxiety, Heart diseases, Clogged blood vessels, a condition medically known as atherosclerosis, High blood cholesterol,

High blood pressure (HBP), Diabetes (high blood sugar level), Obesity and Metabolic syndrome among others.

## How does one test for erectile dysfunction?

Many tests are used to diagnose ED. Some are physical, and some are psychological. Physical examinations, blood tests and urinalysis are carried out among other tests.

## Can I overcome erectile dysfunction?

Sure! There is hope for you. By following the different methods discussed in his book, you can overcome erectile dysfunction.

## Now that I have ED what do I do?

First thing to do is to accept that you have a challenge and open up to your doctor, then you would probably go for a test as explained here

# Frequently Asked Questions

# Index

# Q

# R

# S

# T

## U

## V

## Y

# Photo Credits

Page 3, Изображения пользователя Anton Estrada via Canva.com (Canva Pro License)

https://www.canva.com/photos/MAEgPO73A3g-depressed-man-sitting-on-bed-in-an-empty-room-this-is-major-depressive-disorder/

Page 14, Rido via Canva.com (Canva Pro License)

https://www.canva.com/photos/MABzIeQvptg-sexual-problem-concept/

Page 22, Elnur via Canva.com (Canva Pro License)

https://www.canva.com/photos/MADGrQPIv6I-woman-and-man-in-the-bedroom-during-conflict/

Page 28, Alexander's Images via Canva.com (Canva Pro License)

https://www.canva.com/photos/MAEaOaPgYDc-man-with-dysfunction-problems-doctor-appointment-closeup/

Page 45, Comstock via Canva.com (Canva Pro License)

https://www.canva.com/photos/MAC77pUeZ4E-man-exercising/

Page 92, Elnur via Canva.com (Canva Pro License)

https://www.canva.com/photos/MADFrvIb-fw-the-young-family-discussing-personal-problems/

Page 117, SHOTPRIME via Canva.com (Canva Pro License)

https://www.canva.com/photos/MAC-_gQUW34-man-visiting-his-therapist/

Page 128, KatarzynaBialasiewicz via Canva.com (Canva Pro License)

https://www.canva.com/photos/MADAd8qPG7M-lack-of-sleep/

# References

Colleen M. Story 2021, Healthline, accessed 5 December 2021, https://www.healthline.com/health/erectile-dysfunction/ed-natural-treatments

Charles Patrick Davis, MD, PhD 2021, OnHealth, accessed 5 December 2021, https://www.onhealth.com/content/1/erectile_dysfunction_ed

Cleveland Clinic 2019, accessed 8 December 2021, https://my.clevelandclinic.org/health/diseases/10035-erectile-dysfunction

Dr. Rany Shamloul, MD 2012, The Lancet, accessed 8 December 2021, https://www.thelancet.com/journals/lancet/article/PIIS0140-6736(12)60520-0/fulltext

Edward David Kim, MD, FACS 2020, Medscape, accessed 22 December 2021, https://emedicine.medscape.com/article/444220-overview

Familydoctor.org 2020, accessed 5 December 2021, https://familydoctor.org/condition/erectile-dysfunction/

Harvard Health Publishing 2020, accessed 26 December 2021, https://www.health.harvard.edu/mens-health/5-natural-ways-to-overcome-erectile-dysfunction

Health Direct 2020, accessed 5 December 2021, https://www.healthdirect.gov.au/erectile-dysfunction

Healthy Male n.d, accessed 5 December 2021, https://www.healthymale.org.au/mens-health/erectile-dysfunction

Hims & Hers Health, Inc 2021, accessed 5 December 2021, https://www.forhims.com/blog/erectile-dysfunction-symptoms-causes-treatments

Irvin H. Hirsch , MD 2020, MSD Manual, accessed 5 December 2021,
https://www.msdmanuals.com/professional/genitourinary-
disorders/male-sexual-dysfunction/erectile-dysfunction

Jenny Lelwica Buttaccio, OTR/L 2021, Verywell Health, accessed 5
December 2021, https://www.verywellhealth.com/erectile-dysfunction-
signs-symptoms-and-complications-4160525

John Hopkins Medicine n.d, accessed 8 December
2021, https://www.hopkinsmedicine.org/health/conditions-and-
diseases/erectile-dysfunction

Julie Marks 2020, Everyday Health, accessed 5 December 2021,
https://www.everydayhealth.com/erectile-dysfunction/

Mayo Clinic n.d, accessed 5 December
2021, https://www.mayoclinic.org/diseases-conditions/erectile-
dysfunction/symptoms-causes/syc-20355776

MedlinePlus n.d, accessed 8 December 2021,
https://medlineplus.gov/erectiledysfunction.html

MedStar Health n.d, accessed 8 December 2021,
https://www.medstarhealth.org/services/erectile-dysfunction-ed

Nazia Q Bandukwala, DO 2021, Webmd, accessed 22 December 2021,
https://www.webmd.com/erectile-dysfunction/ss/erectile-dysfunction

National Institute of Diabetes and Digestive and Kidney Diseases n.d,
NIH, accessed 8 December 2021, https://www.niddk.nih.gov/health-
information/urologic-diseases/erectile-dysfunction/symptoms-causes

Rush University Medical Center n.d, accessed 5 December 2021,
https://www.rush.edu/conditions/erectile-dysfunction

The University of Utah Health 2021, accessed 5 December 2021,
https://healthcare.utah.edu/healthfeed/postings/2021/01/top-5-common-
erectile-dysfunction-causes.php

Urology Care Foundation 2018, accessed 26 December 2021,
https://www.urologyhealth.org/urology-a-z/e/erectile-dysfunction-(ed)

Yale Medicine n.d, accessed 26 December 2021,
https://www.yalemedicine.org/conditions/erectile-dysfunction

www.ingramcontent.com/pod-product-compliance
Lightning Source LLC
Chambersburg PA
CBHW060854280326
41934CB00007B/1042